101 Careers in Nursing

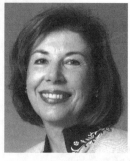

Jeanne M. Novotny, PhD, RN, FAAN, is Dean and Professor at Fairfield University School of Nursing, Fairfield, Connecticut. Her career encompasses more than 3 decades of leadership in nursing education and administration. Dr. Novotny was formerly the Frank Talbott, Jr. Visiting Professor at the University of Virginia; Assistant Dean at the Frances Payne Bolton School of Nursing, Case Western Reserve University, Cleveland, Ohio; and Associate Professor at Kent State University School of Nursing. She received her BSN from The Ohio State University, her MS in Nursing from The Ohio State University, and her PhD in Education from Kent State University. She is a member of the Connecticut Nurses Association/ American Nurses Association and Sigma Theta Tau.

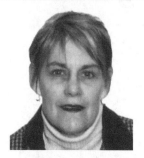

Doris Troth Lippman, APRN, EdD, CS, is a Professor of Nursing at Fairfield University School of Nursing. She also practices as an Advanced Practice Registered Nurse at Fairfield Community Services in Fairfield, Connecticut. Dr. Lippman received her BSN from Cornell University, her MA from Fairfield University, and her MEd and EdD from Columbia University. She is the President-elect of the Connecticut Nurses Association. She is a former member of STTI's Research Committee, and past president of Delta Mu, Yale University's STTI chapter.

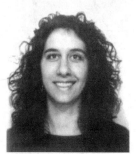

Nicole K. Sanders, BSN, RN, is a staff nurse at Bellevue Hospital, NY, NY. She received a BS degree in Art from the University of Wisconsin-Madison and in 2002 received a BSN from New York University. While a student at NYU she worked as a research assistant for the Nursing Care Quality Initiative, a collaborative project through Mount Sinai NYU Health and the North Shore-Long Island Jewish Health Systems.

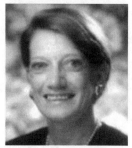

Joyce J. Fitzpatrick, PhD, MBA, RN, FAAN, is the Elizabeth Brooks Ford Professor of Nursing, Frances Payne Bolton School of Nursing, Case Western Reserve University (CWRU) in Cleveland, Ohio where she was Dean from 1982 through 1997. She has received numerous honors and awards including the *American Journal of Nursing* Book of the Year Award 18 times. She is senior editor of the *Annual Review of Nursing Research* series, now in its 21st volume, and editor of the National League for Nursing journal, *Nursing Education Perspectives*. Dr. Fitzpatrick has provided consultation on nursing education and research throughout the world, including universities and health ministries in Africa, Asia, Australia, Europe, Latin America, and the Middle East.

101 Careers in Nursing

Jeanne M. Novotny, PhD, RN, FAAN
Doris T. Lippman, EdD, APRN, CS
Nicole K. Sanders, BSN, RN
Joyce J. Fitzpatrick, PhD, MBA, RN, FAAN
Editors

 Springer Publishing Company

Springer Publishing Company, Inc.
536 Broadway
New York, NY 10012-3955

Acquisitions Editor: Ruth Chasek
Production Editor: Pam Lankas
Cover design by Joanne E. Honigman

04 05 06 07 / 5 4

Library of Congress Cataloging-in-Publication Data

101 careers in nursing / Jeanne M. Novotny . . . [et al.].
     p. ; cm.
   Includes bibliographical references and index.
   ISBN 0-8261-2014-8
   1. Nursing—Vocational guidance—United States.   I. Title: One hundred and one careers in nursing.   II. Novotny, Jeanne.
   [DNLM: 1. Career Choice. 2. Nursing. WY 16 Z999 2003]
   RT82.A15 2003
   610.73'06'9—dc21   2003050615

Printed in the United States of America by Maple-Vail Book Manufacturing Group.

In memory of Joette Clark,
who inspired many nurses in their careers.

Contents

Contributor

Tracey E. Robert, MA, LPC, NCCC, is a licensed professional counselor and a nationally certified counselor with a designated career specialty. She is a principal in the career-development firm Tracey Robert Associates of Fairfield, providing career counseling and consulting to individuals and organizations. She has more than 20 years experience in career and life planning and adult development. Robert has provided career development and relocation consulting and counseling for many varied corporate clients.

Robert's background includes experience in the manufacturing, health care, and educational services fields. She holds a master's degree in counseling from Fairfield University and a B.A. from Dunbarton College. She is a doctoral candidate in counselor education specializing in community counseling. Her research involves work and spirituality.

Introduction

*Jeanne M. Novotny, Joyce J. Fitzpatrick,
and Doris T. Lippman*

Nursing is the health care career of the 21st century. The nation's nursing shortage is projected to worsen significantly over the next 2 decades. According to the Department of Health and Human Services, there were an estimated 1,189 million registered nurses working in the United States in 2000, with the demand for nurses estimated at 2 million. This translates to a 6% shortage of nurses. Based on what is known about trends in the supply of registered nurses and the anticipated demand, the shortage is expected to double to 12% by 2010, to triple by 2015, and continue growing to 29% by 2020. Nursing is listed everywhere as one of the top growth professions.

If you are reading this book, you are undoubtedly a college-bound student with ambition and the desire to work with people, or a nurse who is interested in changing your career focus. We applaud your interest in, curiosity about, and commitment to a career in nursing. Nursing is a discipline that offers both a lifetime of satisfaction in service to others and rewards so great that they cannot be measured. In addition, the choices of careers are, at minimum, 101 possibilities! Can you name one other career path that can take you in so many directions? This means that as you grow and develop as a person you can continually reinvent who you are as a professional nurse. When you choose to become a nurse you will know that at the end of each day you have done work that is substantial and meaningful. You will have opportunities to work with people of all ages in environments that range from caring for a patient who is critically ill to being an editor of a nursing journal.

The purpose of this book is to show you the possibilities inherent in the profession. Use it as you would use a reference book and select those areas that interest you.

It is important to note some of the following as you decide your career path. Old ways of surviving in the workplace are obsolete. Nurses are becoming increasingly aware that as they navigate a career the focus needs to be on the opportunities rather than on what are perceived as deficits. It also is important to be as clear as possible in your career goal and to focus on the positive aspects of the work. Health care is changing and so are the skills needed to have a long and productive career as a professional nurse. When a business changes so do the characteristics of the individuals who survive and thrive in a new environment. This is why nurses engage in learning on a continuous basis.

Employers want a health care professional who is self-motivated, shows initiative, has an inner drive for doing well, and is optimistic enough to weather the daily fluctuations in job satisfaction. Professionals who are alert to the new opportunities that change creates are sought throughout the health care system. Nurses have had a long and rich history of responding to change with hope and possibility for the future.

Your career is your business. You must think of patients as your customers. You must be a steward of the resources of your employer just as if the time, equipment, and money are your own and you are the owner of the business. You must rely on your self and at the same time collaborate with others. Seeking continuing education and earning a baccalaureate degree or advanced degree are ways to give you the competitive edge in the marketplace. You will be resilient to change if you are self-aware and have self-control, if you have motivation and empathy, and if you have leadership and communication skills.

This book is a directory of careers that will give you an idea of the infinite opportunities available no matter where your interests are focused. Use this book as you would use a dictionary. As you read and search various entries, match the nursing career with what your interests are in general and how you see yourself spending time as your life evolves. Keep asking yourself, "What would I like to be doing in the future?" and then set goals and develop a plan. Develop a plan that is flexible, but also serves as a road map.

In addition to the 101 different careers cited, a number of nurses in cutting-edge fields are profiled. You will read about them in their own words and find out why their careers are so meaningful. These nurses share their ideas and beliefs about their specific careers in nursing. Each of these profiles will give you a sense of the opportunities inherent in a nursing career choice.

Always keep motivated by using your inner self to move and guide you toward new and fresh goals and ideas. Take initiative and strive to improve and to persevere in the face of setbacks and frustrations. Be confident, take steps to develop your career, and take pride in accomplishments.

We hope that this book will encourage those thinking about a career in nursing to get started, to those in the field to stay and reinvent themselves if necessary, and to those retiring to encourage them to stay connected to the profession. Nursing is the translation of knowledge into human caring. What better way could you spend your life?

Acute Care Nurse Practitioner

1. **Basic description**—Acute care nurse practitioners are advanced practice nurses who specialize in providing care for acutely ill patients in a variety of settings. The environment in which acute care nurse practitioners function is very intense and dramatic. Some of the characteristics of the work include coordinating patient care, assessing the patient's health history, ordering diagnostic tests, performing therapeutic procedures, and prescribing medications. Possibilities to work exist in:
   - Emergency rooms
   - Operating rooms
   - Critical care units
   - Transplant units

2. **Educational requirements**—MSN with advanced practice certification as an Acute Care Nurse Practitioner. Graduate programs are generally 2 years in length. The number of schools that offer this specialty is limited, therefore entry into these programs is competitive.

3. **Core competencies/skills needed:**
   - Technical competency involving use of complex and computerized equipment
   - Regulating ventilators
   - Hemodynamic monitoring
   - Obtaining blood samples from central IV lines
   - Interpersonal competency dealing with patients and their families in life-threatening situations
   - Ability to work with interdisciplinary teams
   - Extensive experience and expertise in assessing and managing acutely ill patients

4. **Compensation**—Salaries vary according to place of employment and geographic location. The average is $62,000–$80,000, but can be much higher depending on level of responsibility.

5. **Employment outlook**—Moderate
6. **Related Web sites and professional organizations:**
   - American Association of Nurse Practitioners: www.aanp.org
   - Nurse Practitioner Support Services: www.nurse.net
   - Cost and Quality: The Emergence of the Acute Care Nurse Practitioner: www.cost-quality.com
   - Nurse Practitioner Associates for Continuing Education: www.npace.org
   - American Nurses Association Credentialing Center: www.ana.org

---

Addictions Counselor

1. **Basic description**—Nurses who are addictions counselors work in organizations that specialize in helping clients overcome addictive disorders. Treatment programs exist in all regions of the country. Chemical dependency is a major health problem and nurses work with clients to help them learn more effective ways of coping.
2. **Educational requirements**—BSN is preferred with certification as a Certified Addictions Registered Nurse (CARN). CARN is a specialty licensure required beyond the RN level specific to working as an Addictions Specialist. Three years' experience as a registered nurse is necessary. Within the 5 years prior to the application for certification, a minimum of 4,000 hours (2 years) of nursing experience related to addictions is required. There is also an advanced practice certification that requires the MSN.
3. **Core competencies/skills needed:**
   - Excellent interpersonal and counseling skills
   - Good interviewing techniques

- Strong assessment skills
- Counseling ability
- Compassion and empathy
- Interest in mental health
- Ability to work in interdisciplinary teams

4. **Compensation**—Varies with place of employment and geographic location; the average is $30,000 to $35,000, but is often higher depending on certification and level of responsibility.

5. **Employment outlook**—Moderate

6. **Related Web sites and professional organizations:**
   - International Nurses Society on Addictions: www.intnsa.org
   - American Nurses Association Peer Assistance Program: www.ana.org

---

Administrator/Manager

1. **Basic description**—Nurse administrators and executive directors are needed in numerous organizations. Knowledge of finance, law, human resources, and related topics improve the systems necessary for the advancement of health care administration and delivery. Nurses are managers, administrators, and executive directors in hospitals, nursing homes, colleges and universities, and health maintenance organizations. Administrators employ, direct, evaluate, promote, and terminate employees. An administrator must have the ability to analyze budgets and make certain that financial plans are consistent with organizational mission and goals. Work hours are often long, but the rewards are gratifying in shaping the future of the organization, the delivery of care, and the profession.

2. **Educational requirements**—BSN is now the entry-level degree. The majority of high-level nursing executives hold an MSN or

an MBA. In addition, many nurse executives are certified in administration through the American Nurses Association Credentialing Center.

3. **Core competencies/skills needed:**
    - Human resource knowledge
    - Excellent interpersonal skills
    - Ability to communicate clearly and persuasively
    - Leadership skills
    - Self-confidence
    - Budgeting and finance skills
    - Writing skills
    - Strong work ethic
    - Managerial competencies

4. **Compensation**—Salaries vary according to place of employment and geographic location, and the type of organization, whether it is national or local, and the level of the administrative position. The average range is between $80,000 and $120,000.

5. **Employment outlook**—Moderate

6. **Related Web sites and professional organizations:**
    - American Organization of Nurse Executives (AONE): www.aone.org
    - American Nurses Association (ANA): www.ana.org
    - American College of Healthcare Executives: www.ache.org

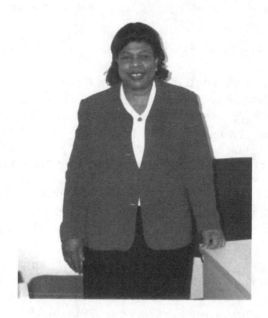

Lorna Green, Nurse Manager.

An Interview with Lorna Green, Nurse Manager, Gero-Psychiatric Unit

What is your educational background in nursing (and other areas) and what formal credentials do you hold?

My name is Lorna Victoria Green and I am a clinical nurse manager at Mount Sinai Hospital in New York City. I have been employed at Mount Sinai for the past 23 years. My experience includes 9 years as a general duty psychiatric nurse, working with geriatrics, adult, and adolescent patients with various psychiatric diagnoses and symptoms/

behaviors, 2 years as senior clinical nurse, and 12 years as a clinical nurse manager.

My credentials include associate degree (Nursing) from Borough of Manhattan Community College in 1981; a bachelor of science (Nursing) cum laude from Medgar Evers College in 1990; and a master of science (Nursing) from Hunter College in 1998.

How did you first become interested in your current career?

For as long as I can remember, I wanted to be a nurse. During my early childhood, I saw my mother, aunts, and neighborhood women minister to friends and relatives who became ill. They provided whatever care was needed for as long as it was needed, without payment or other expectations. All care was rendered at home. Only one doctor was available to provide care for all the people on our island and the nearest hospital was only accessible by boat or by small plane in the later years. Without the diagnosis, care, and support of the neighbors, friends, and relatives, many people would have suffered and died. Therefore, I do not think that I ever "became interested" in nursing, I believe that I was born into it. How fortunate for me that my family, culture, and circumstances of birth allowed me to recognize and develop my passion at a young age. It would not be an exaggeration to state that nursing is not only my profession, it is truly my vocation and one of the most important reasons I am on this earth.

What are the most rewarding aspects of your career?

Every day in nursing is rewarding in some way for me. Specifically, though, one of the most rewarding days in my life is the day I assumed responsibility of the geriatric psychiatry unit. The unit presented a myriad of challenges. Among the most difficult was its reputation for not being consumer oriented and the lack of cohesiveness among staff. Interpersonal relationships were fraught with conflict at times. I am proud to say that through hard work and compromise, we have turned the unit around. We now frequently receive complimentary letters from patients and their families. Doctors, nurses, and other staff members have voiced their appreciation for the improved environment. I take great pride and personal fulfillment in my contributions and continually work hard to seek further enhancements to achieve total consumer and staff satisfaction.

Describe a typical workday in your current job.

I believe that a "typical workday" does not exist in nursing because we are dealing with human beings who are unique and are experiencing illness, emotional stressors, and/or disorders of some variety and we are involved with the client's family members, living situations, after-care, and concurrent medical problems. Thus, we must be able to switch gears and adapt on a moment's notice.

An overview of my daily schedule usually includes the following:

Check e-mail and voicemail upon arrival to the office

Make patient rounds with staff on both units

Perform environmental rounds with primary goal of ensuring safety of furniture/equipment and other patient safety issues

Participate in the morning interdisciplinary treatment team meeting

Sit in on patient group activities

Perform incident investigations

Assess and respond to patient/family/staff/union issues

Assess and evaluate for response to care rendered

Evaluate and counsel staff, provide in-services

Resolve budget/staffing/scheduling issues

Assist with program development

Communicate with peer nurse managers, care center director, and other hospital staff on a daily basis

Attend off-unit meetings covering topics such as special review and performance improvement, and attend leadership meetings with my director of nursing or with my senior vice president of nursing

Perform other duties such as participating as co-chair of the Professional Practice Committee and being involved as a member of the management team for the negotiation of the employment contract

Provide leadership to maintain harmony with an ultimate goal of consumer and staff satisfaction

What advice would you give to someone contemplating the same career path in nursing?

The most important advice I would impart to a nurse considering a career in administration/management would be to spend the time at the bedside involved in direct patient care as a staff nurse to broaden your knowledge base and gain perspective. Do not jump into the leadership role prematurely. The more you experience and develop, the greater amount of resource will be available to you when you take on additional responsibilities in a leadership role and this will boost your confidence level and others confidence in you when you are making critical decisions.

How do you balance career and other aspects of your life?

As mentioned earlier, nursing is not my career, it is my vocation. I am able to have a full life because of nursing, not despite nursing. When at the hospital, I give my full attention to my patients, their families/ friends, my staff, my peers, my boss, and other hospital personnel. My children have grown up with a mother who is a nurse, therefore, like I understood my mother, they have learned to accept that my responsibilities are an important part of who I am. I also am able to achieve greater gratification from my children, my home, and outside activities because I am happy in my role as a clinical nurse manager at Mount Sinai Hospital.

Adult Nurse Practitioner

1. **Basic description**—Adult nurse practitioners are advanced practice nurses who specialize in providing primary care to adults in a variety of settings, such as hospitals, outpatient clinics, ambulatory care settings, physicians' offices, community-based clinics, and health care agencies. The adult nurse practitioner functions as a primary care provider and focuses on maintaining health and wellness in acute and chronic illnesses. Some of the characteristics of the work are:
    *   Teaching patients to manage chronic conditions
    *   Assessing the patient's health history and status
    *   Ordering diagnostic tests
    *   Performing therapeutic procedures
    *   Prescribing medications
2. **Educational requirements**—MSN with advanced practice certification as an Adult Nurse Practitioner. Graduate programs are generally 2 years in length.
3. **Core competencies/skills needed:**
    *   Health assessment skills
    *   Interpersonal skills
    *   Ability to work in interdisciplinary teams
    *   Knowledge of acute and chronic diseases
    *   Health promotion knowledge and skills
    *   Knowledge of primary care provider role
    *   Must possess extensive experience and expertise in assessing and managing patients in primary care settings
4. **Compensation**—Salaries vary according to place of employment and geographic location. The average is $62,000 to $80,000.
5. **Employment Outlook**—High

6. **Related Web sites and professional organizations:**
   • American Association of Nurse Practitioners: www.aanp.org
   • Nurse Practitioner Support Services: www.nurse.net
   • Nurse Practitioner Associates for Continuing Education: www.npace.org
   • American Nurses Association Credentialing Center: www.ana.org
   • Nurse Practitioner Programs Directory: www.allnursingschools.com

---

Ambulatory Care/Health Center Nurse

1. **Basic description**—An ambulatory care nurse or health center nurse works as part of a multidisciplinary health care team to provide primary care to a specific population. Depending on the role the nurse plays within the health center, the work activities will differ. A triage nurse may primarily work in a walk-in area or on the telephone assessing the patients and making determinations on the priority with which they must be seen or referred. Working with a multidisciplinary team entails gathering a medical history and information about the chief complaint and checking vital signs. Once the practitioner has seen the patient, the nurse will perform follow-up treatment such as drawing labs and teaching the patient regarding the condition and discharge instructions.

2. **Educational requirements**—RN preparation.

3. **Core competencies/skills needed:**
   • Knowledge of illnesses and symptoms including diagnosis and management
   • Experience with triage

- Strong assessment and organizational skills
- Communication skills
- Ability to collaborate and function as a member of a multidisciplinary team
- Ability to function in a fast-paced environment
- Interest in working with a diverse population

4. **Compensation**—Varies according to place of employment and geographic location.

5. **Employment outlook**—High

6. **Related Web site and professional organization:**
   - American Academy of Ambulatory Care Nursing: www.aaacn.org/

Armed Services Nurse

1. **Basic description**—Nurses in the Army, Navy, and Air Force provide quality care in both inpatient and outpatient settings to the men and women on active duty and to their families. Armed Services nurses may be called for wartime duty, sent overseas for service, or placed in a combat hospital. Characteristics of the work are broad and cut across all nursing roles.

   Examples of settings where they work include the following:
   - Ambulatory clinics
   - Community hospitals
   - Medical centers
   - Hospital ships
   - Aircraft
   - Field hospitals

2. **Educational requirements**—BSN with RN licensure required for active duty. Candidates must meet the requirements for an officer in the Army, Navy, or Air Force and be accepted into that

military branch. U.S. citizenship is required. A large percentage of nurses in the armed services have graduate degrees; thus, they are eligible for higher ranks and higher pay.

3. **Core competencies/skills needed:**
   - Leadership skills
   - Strong interpersonal skills
   - Maturity
   - Excellent physical and emotional health
   - Flexible regarding time and geographic location
   - Willingness to be called to wartime duty
   - Able to work in a structure environment

4. **Compensation**—Salaries range between $40,000 and $45,000 at the entry level. Benefits include living expenses, education, and more. Retirement is based on 20 years of service. The opportunity exists to change jobs without losing seniority, and in addition, candidates have a chance to serve their country.

5. **Employment outlook**—High

6. **Related Web sites and professional organizations:**
   - Army: www.army.mil/
   - Navy: www.navy.mil/
   - Air Force: www.airforce.mil/

An Interview with
Ella Bradshaw,
Armed Services Nurse

What is your educational background in nursing (and other areas) and what formal credentials do you hold?

I obtained a bachelor of science degree in Nursing, May 1980, at George-town University; a master of science degree in Health Care Administration, May 1997, at the University of New Haven; a master of science Nursing, dual degree, Medical Surgical Nursing and Nursing Administration in May 1999, at the University of Maryland; and a post master's certificate as Family Nurse Practitioner in December 2002, from the University of Maryland.

How did you first become interested in your current career?

My initial attention to nursing occurred when I was in junior high school during a time when a family member became ill and was hospitalized for a short period of time prior to his death. The nurses provided such empathetic care to both the patient and my entire family that I began to think this was something I would like to do. I thought about it for a brief time but never really looked into how to become a nurse. During my senior year of high school, I realized that I had to apply to colleges and I needed a major, so I applied to nursing school. Upon completing nursing school, I started working at George Washington University Medical Center on an internal medicine ward and really liked what I was doing. The patients were very sick but I liked caring for them and their families. The work was hard and very tiring but I seemed to have a source of energy and enthusiasm for the profession of nursing, and I came to love what I was doing.

After working at GW for just over 3 years I decided that I wanted to do something different in nursing so I joined the military. My initial contract was for 3 years, and since I had already worked for 3 years I knew exactly what that period of time would mean in the scheme of my life. In September 1983, I joined the military and began an adventure. Being a military nurse encompasses two roles: first as a military officer, then as a nurse. Being educated as a nurse and working as a nurse made it a bit difficult initially for me to envision myself as a military officer first then a nurse. I quickly learned that being in the military would offer tremendous challenge and growth in both roles. The opportunities for me as a military officer have been unending in terms of administrative, leadership and management, educational, and clinical experiences.

My love is medical surgical nursing but I have worked in obstetrics, psychiatry, orthopedics, cardiology, gynecology (all inpatient), and a number of ambulatory care centers. I have had various levels of administrative and leadership positions in addition to clinical positions. These experiences were all available without me having to change employers, and the preparation for the positions is a natural part of my career track in the military. There is a strong commitment to training and education, and these opportunities are available to all.

As a military nurse my relationships with the patients and their families are different from when I was a nurse in the civilian community. Being in the military makes me more than a professional nurse; it makes me a member of the same community as the patients and the families I care for. I am better able to understand their needs for medical care, administrative issues, social issues, stressors related to the job in general, deployment or unique work environments, and so forth, because I face the same issues as they do. I know what it takes to help an active duty member get well and get back to work. The relationship is a much closer working relationship and the contributions that I make can be enormous. Military nursing is global and I have formed networks worldwide and no matter what, I know that I belong to a community. I believe that joining the military was one of the best decisions I have ever made and I highly recommend military nursing as a career to anyone with an interest in nursing.

What are the most rewarding aspects of your career?

The military is committed to training and education and I have been on the giving and receiving end of both. I discovered that I really enjoy teaching and for many years I have been able to work with new personnel and help them transition into the military health care system. I have had the privilege of working with both corpsman (medical technicians) and nurses, teaching them their role and the skills necessary for their position in health care. I am always astounded as I watch these individuals acquire the clinical skills and attitudes required to provide excellent care the patients. This is a fabulous opportunity to teach people the true value of nursing, to work with individuals new to the profession and help them understand what it is about nursing they love (or will come to love) and how they can translate it into practice.

There are numerous committees and command function teams to participate in, so I have had the opportunity to influence nursing practice through different committees. I have been actively involved in Standards and Practice Committees, JCAHO function teams, Peer Review, and Ethics Committees for most of my career. My goal is to remain current in education and practice by researching practice issues and writing practice guidelines, Thus I will be able to keep colleagues current in their practice. There is an expectation that as you become more senior in your career, you will shape the practice so you are introduced to committees and command function teams early so you get an experience you can build on. I have been afforded the opportunity to work across clinical and administrative lines and learn about how decisions are made at the highest level. In talking and with many of my civilian friends, they have not been afforded the same opportunities.

Describe a typical workday in your current job.

My current position is Director, Nurse Intern Program. The nurse intern program is a 13-week internship for new Navy nurses reporting to Bethesda. The program consists of 11 weeks of clinical rotation through medical surgical areas and outpatient through clinics, and 2 weeks of classroom instruction. The clinical rotations are designed to facilitate the new nurses in understanding the role and responsibilities of nurses in the different settings. The didactic material covers both clinical and administrative topics such as physical assessment, clinical decision-making skills, conflict management, effective communication, organizational structure, management of enlisted personnel, skills workshop, and a medical surgical course (1 week long approved for 43.2 CEUs). The new Navy nurses must learn their role as military officer and registered nurse and this internship helps with the transition to both roles.

My role includes working in the various clinical areas with the new nurses teaching them direct hands on care of patients along with all the administrative issues that go along with providing the care. I instruct and evaluate their clinical skills, organizational skills and time management, interactions with various levels of staff, involvement in multidisciplinary teams, and provide an orientation plan to the nurse manager of the unit when they are assigned to a permanent workspace.On days when the nurses are off, I work on administrative matters, which could include anything from licensure issues for the new nurses (we receive graduate nurses from all over the country who have not taken their nursing boards and their issues are different depending on the state where they are seeking licensure), information about deployment, obtaining legal information pertinent to deployment, clinical practice issues, and curriculum development. I develop the curriculum for the didactic programs offered to the new nurses as well as other educational programs offered through staff education. I also teach many of the topics offered through these programs.

What advice would you give to someone contemplating the same career path in nursing?

I love nursing and I find it to be very rewarding but I have done many different things in nursing. Nursing can be very hard work but it is very challenging and there are numerous opportunities for growth if one takes the time to look. I have chosen to remain clinical and I like bedside nursing but I have mixed various experiences in my career to provide clinical, administrative, and personal growth for myself. My rewards are internal and I enjoy what I do. I live with the possibility of being deployed and being separated from my family, but military nursing is what I do and who I am. My advice would be to do your homework: investigate the full scope of nursing, look for all the things that might be possible, then think about who you are and what you really want to achieve and go for it. Nursing offers a large variety of opportunities to anyone who is flexible and willing to try new things. The military offers tremendous opportunities (clinical, management and leadership, education) and there are sacrifices, but if you are flexible you can certainly be successful.

How do you balance career and other aspects of your life?

As a nurse in the military it is extremely important for me to be able to balance my personal life and my professional life. Nursing has always been very rewarding to me but I put in a lot of very long hours and there are many days when I am absolutely exhausted but I always think of the positive impact for patients and their family and this makes everything seem worthwhile. I concentrate on my own family when I am not at work and my goal is to do something as a family that will be enjoyable for us all. I plan fun time into my off-duty time and I plan for periods of relaxation. I like traveling and I plan trips at least twice a year. Recently, I have been working full time and going to graduate school full time, and I realized that I was not spending enough time with my family. School was a goal, something I felt I needed to do at the time and I was able to balance school, work, and home until my last semester when I realized that school had practically become my whole life. As soon as school was finished, I started spending more time with my family and planning personal time for us. I make it a priority to do fun things when I am not working and not to sit around resting up for my next block of workdays.

Now with the threat of war and the possibility of deployment, it is more important than ever for me to take care of myself and be clear about what my needs are at this very time. I know that it is so easy to become consumed with the demands of a busy successful career so I always have to remind myself that I must take care of me personally so that I can continue to take care of others. I have learned over the years to plan and write out goals with realistic time lines. When I was first exploring the option of graduate school, the most important question for me was "what can I realistically accomplish during this period" while working full-time. I wanted to be a nurse practitioner but I did not have time to complete the required clinical hours, so I went to school for health care administration because I have an interest in managed care and my career and personal life would allow me time to complete this track. Since then I have attended another graduate program (paid for by the military) and a post master's program at times when these programs fit into my life. I try to be realistic about what I can accomplish and what I am willing to sacrifice knowing that I want to have a successful career and a happy family. With every decision I make I must consider both career and family, and decide what the impact will be for me personally.

Most recently I have people commenting that "I don't appear to be upset about the impending deployment." My perspective is that I might be going somewhere whether or not I'm upset, so while I'm here I need to continue to do the job I do daily and make sure I take care of myself personally and enjoy my family for as long as I can. Being in the military is what I do, it is my choice, and if called to action I am ready.

Attorney

1. **Basic description**—Nurse attorneys engage in a range of legal activities including the following:
   - Provide legal consult/prosecute/defend cases; may represent individuals, patients, health professionals or institutions.
   - Provide depositions and court testimony.
   - Engage in legal research.
   - Define standards of care.
   - Serve as quality-of-care experts for hospitals and other health care institutions.
   - Review cases.
   - Define applicable standards of care.
   - Organize records.
   - Research the literature.
   - Provide behind-the-scenes or up-front consultations.
   - Interview clients and witnesses.
   - Prepare exhibits.
   - Prepare questions for depositions and court.
2. **Educational requirements**—RN preparation, JD degree.
3. **Core competencies/skills needed:**
   - Logical thinking skills
   - Knowledge of judicial system and health care legislation
4. **Compensation**—Varies with the place of employment, ranges from an average beginning salary of $60,000 to more than $200,000 if employed in a major law firm.
5. **Employment outlook**—Moderate
6. **Related Web sites and professional organizations:**
   - The American Association of Nurse Attorneys (TAANA): www.taana.org
   - Registered Nurse Experts, Inc.: www.rnexperts.com

Author/Writer

1. **Basic description**—RN who works in any area of writing. This written material may be used in research, biomedical research, education, training, sales and marketing, and other medical mediums and communication forms. The work can be tedious and isolating. Writers need the ability at times to work with voluminous technical information. Authors or editors may write for medical and general interest publications, freelance, professional organizations, and medical trade journals.

2. **Educational requirements**—RN preparation; BSN or higher often required.

3. **Core competencies/skills needed:**
   - Good command of the English language
   - Ability to work alone
   - Ability to meet deadlines
   - Excellent writing skills
   - Health care–related knowledge

4. **Compensation**—Varies with the type of writing; range is considerable.

5. **Employment opportunities**—High

6. **Related Web sites and professional organizations:**
   - Registered Nurse Experts, Inc.: www.rnexperts.com
   - Tips to get published: www.medi-smart.com/authors.htm
   - American Medical Writers Association: www.amwa.org

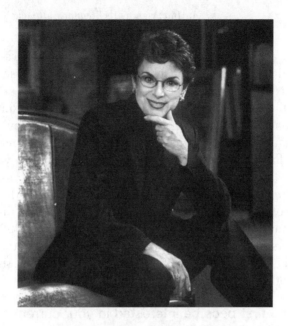

Eleanor Sullivan, Nurse Author.

An Interview with Eleanor Sullivan, Nurse Author

What is your educational background in nursing (and other areas) and what formal credentials do you hold?

I consider myself a nurse author with experience both in nursing and in writing. Following several clinical and teaching positions, I became associate dean of nursing at the University of Missouri–St. Louis and later at the University of Minnesota before becoming dean of the School of Nursing at the University of Kansas, as well as president of the nursing honor society, Sigma Theta Tau International. I have also served on the board of directors of the American Association of Colleges of

Nursing, on an advisory council at the National Institutes of Health, and I helped in the successful lobbying efforts to establish a nursing institute at NIH, among others.

I have published several award-winning textbooks, including *Effective Leadership and Management in Nursing* (Prentice Hall), now in its fifth edition, and more than 40 articles in scientific and professional journals. *Becoming Influential: A Guide for Nurses*, my latest book, was recently released by Prentice Hall. From 1997 to 2002 I was editor of the *Journal of Professional Nursing*, the official publication of the American Association of Colleges of Nursing. Recently I have turned my attention to writing mystery fiction. My credentials include: a PhD from St. Louis University, a MSN in psychiatric nursing from Southern Illinois University at Edwardsville, a BSN from St. Louis University, and an ADN from St. Louis Community College.

How did you first become interested in your current career?

I wrote my first nursing book, *Effective Leadership and Management in Nursing*, because few nursing management books included content from organizational and management literature. The book was a runaway best-seller; I am currently working on the sixth edition.

After publishing several more nursing books, numerous scientific and professional articles, and editing a professional journal for several years, I decided to try my hand at writing a mystery. I thought it might be fun to create a story using a nurse sleuth and portraying nursing realistically. With my writing background, I thought I could transfer my skills to another genre. I couldn't have been more wrong!

Discovering how difficult it was to create anything that read like published mysteries, I did what any good academic does: I went to the literature, studied books and periodicals, took classes, and attended conferences to learn how to create mystery fiction. Finally, my work was good enough to attract the attention of a publisher.

What are the most rewarding aspects of your career?

I view my writing as an extension of my nursing work. My goal is to share what I have learned with students, nurses, and, now through mystery fiction, with the public. When nurses say my work helped them or that they saw themselves in my fiction, I feel grateful. When people who are not nurses tell me they learned about nursing through my fiction, I feel satisfied that I met my goal.

Also rewarding were my experiences as a dean and as president of Sigma Theta Tau International. During my tenure as dean of the School of Nursing at the University of Kansas, we became a research-funded school, created an endowment, began several programs across the state of Kansas, and received funding for a new nursing education building. As Sigma Theta Tau International president, I helped create our vision for the future, expanded diversity, and increased public attention to nursing. Both of these positions have afforded me opportunities to contribute to the larger good of both nursing and society.

Describe a typical workday in your current job

I am in my office every week day from 9 to 5. I spend most of my time writing either on professional work or mystery fiction. I spend some time on professional meetings and their preparation and on promoting my writing. Regardless, I am always thinking about writing—in my car, exercising, or even in the shower! Then I quickly make notes on whatever I can find. I have even resorted to scribbling on my hand!

What advice would you give to someone contemplating the same career path in nursing?

Writing gives you a chance to express yourself and share your thoughts, ideas, and viewpoint. (Even in fiction you reveal your beliefs whether you intend to or not.) If you want to write, read everything you can, especially in the genre that interests you. Get as much out of every experience you can, preferably making notes on your observations, what happened, and what you learned. Then write, write, write. Get feedback on your work from other writers who are more experienced than you, such as teachers or professional editors. Finally, there is only one way to success as a writer: persistence. Many excellent writers have failed to be published because they gave up. Don't let that be you!

How do you balance career and other aspects of your life?

Since I was widowed with five young children before I entered college, I learned how to manage competing demands for my time. My system is to prioritize, organize, and, most important, to persevere. My latest nursing book, *Becoming Influential: A Guide for Nurses*, explains how to do that.

Do you have any other advice for other nurses who might want to pursue this type of nursing career?

If you are starting out to write, explore your interests. Discover your passion and write about that. Writing is hard work, and you will be living and working with your material a long time. Be sure you love the topic or the genre well enough to sustain you through rewriting, editing, and the process of becoming published. Also, do not count on your writing to support you; few of us do. We do it for the love of it.

Burn Nurse

1. **Basic description**—Nurses who work with burn patients perform comprehensive, highly specialized critical care to adults, geriatric, and pediatric patients who have sustained burn injuries involving up to 100% of total body surface area. The working environment on a burn unit is very intense. The nurse must continually be involved in assessment, planning, and evaluation of care. As part of a highly functioning interdisciplinary team, the nurse must recognize physiological and behavioral changes and know their significance to patient survival. Burn nurses administer pain and other medications, operate special equipment specific to the burn unit, and must maintain fluid and electrolyte balance in their patients.

2. **Educational requirements**—RN preparation.

3. **Core competencies/skills needed**—Most burn units require 1 year of general medical-surgical or critical care experience, as well as the following:
   - Knowledge of the pathophysiology of burns
   - Complete understanding of fluid and electrolyte balance
   - Technical competency involving complex equipment
   - Ability to work with patients on ventilators
   - Knowledge of pain management
   - Skilled in the use of aseptic technique
   - Interpersonal competency dealing with patients and families in life-threatening situations
   - Ability to work with interdisciplinary teams

4. **Compensation**—Similar to nurses in other specialty units such as critical care; starting RN salary is approximately $40,000.

5. **Employment outlook**—High

6. **Related Web sites and professional organizations:**
    *   American Burn Association: www.ameriburn.org
    *   Nurse Friendly: www.nursefriendly.com/burn/

Camp Nurse

1. **Basic description**—A camp nurse provides full health care to children attending camp. In some situations, camps are specific to children with special needs, for example, children with asthma, or children with diabetes. The working environment for a camp nurse is usually one of low stress. Much of the time is spent working with groups of children in an outdoor setting. The work is normally short term during the summer months. However, if a crisis arises the nurse must have the critical care and rapid response background to deal with life-threatening situations.
2. **Educational requirements**—RN preparation.
3. **Core competencies/skills needed**—Camp nurses require knowledge of first aid, cardiopulmonary resuscitation, bee stings, snakebites, cuts, and other acute traumatic episodes. Other requirements include
    *   Understanding separation anxiety
    *   Interpersonal skills
    *   First aid knowledge
    *   Physical and emotional assessment skills
    *   Medication management
    *   Ability to respond to unexpected situations
4. **Compensation**—Varies according to place of employment and geographic location.
5. **Employment outlook**—High
6. **Related Web sites and professional organizations:**
    *   Association of Camp Nurses: www.campnurse.org
    *   Camp Nurse Jobs: www.campnursejobs.com

Cardiovascular Nurse

1. **Basic description**—The nurse with an interest in cardiac or vascular nursing works with patients who have compromised cardiovascular systems. Cardiac nurses perform postoperative care on a surgical unit, stress test evaluations, cardiac monitoring, vascular monitoring, and health assessments. The setting can be varied depending on the focus of the patient population. Cardiac/ vascular nurses can work in acute care settings with surgical patients, outpatient clinics doing case management, and in home care.

2. **Educational requirements**—RN preparation.

3. **Core competencies/skills needed:**
    *   Basic Life Support and Advanced Cardiac Life Support certification
    *   Proficiency in reading cardiac monitors
    *   Critical care experience
    *   Knowledge of cardiac rhythms and cardiac disease
    *   Good interpersonal skills
    *   Ability to work with interdisciplinary teams
    *   Ability to manage acute episodes in chronically ill patients

4. **Compensation**—Varies according to place of employment and geographic setting.

5. **Employment outlook**—High

6. **Related Web sites and professional organizations:**
    *   American Association of Cardiovascular and Pulmonary Rehabilitation: www.aacvpr.org
    *   National Association of Vascular Access Networks: www.navannet.org
    *   Society for Vascular Nursing: www.svnnet.org

Case Manager

1. **Basic description**—Case management is the process of organizing and coordinating resources and services in response to individual health care needs along the illness and care continuum in multiple settings. There are many models for case management given client, context, or setting. The nurse case manager assesses and monitors clients and the health care delivery services that they require. Case management is directed toward a targeted or selected client/family population such as transplant, head-injured, or frail elderly clients. The goals are to center services around the patient, to foster patient self-managed care, and maximize efficient and cost-effective use of health resources. The focus is cost saving and continuity of care. Case managers have the opportunity to work in hospitals, community outreach, clinics, occupational health, insurance companies, and health maintenance organizations.

2. **Educational requirements**—RN preparation; BSN degree; master's degree preferred.

3. **Core competencies/skills needed:**
    *   Strong knowledge base in both the financial and clinical aspects of care
    *   Understanding of community resources
    *   Strong communication skills
    *   Effective skills in managing, teaching, and negotiating
    *   Ability to work with interdisciplinary groups
    *   Ability to focus on patients and families

4. **Compensation**—Varies depending on the place of employment and geographic location.

5. **Employment outlook**—High

6. **Related Web sites and professional organizations:**
   - The American Association of Managed Care Nurses: www.aamcn.org
   - Commission for Case Manager Certification: www.ccmcertification.org
   - Case Management Society of America: www.cmsa.org

Childbirth Educator

1. **Basic description**—The childbirth educator provides informational and educational classes for expectant parents. Classes include information on relaxation techniques, comfort measures, breathing techniques, and birth options. Childbirth educators play an important role in the emotional, physical, and informational support for expectant parents. Most hospitals and birthing centers offer this type of educational program for their clients. Usually a nurse with excellent teaching and interpersonal skills is selected to teach class on site to expectant parents.

2. **Educational requirements**—RN preparation. Certification may be obtained through the Childbirth and Postpartum Professional Association (CAPPA).

3. **Core competencies/skills needed:**
   - Must have knowledge about the childbearing years, pregnancy, and labor and delivery
   - Teaching ability
   - Clinical competence in obstetrical nursing
   - Interpersonal skills
   - Collaboration with physicians

4. **Compensation**—Varies with place of employment and geographic location, and credentials of the childbirth educator.

5. **Employment outlook**—Moderate

6. **Related Web sites and professional organizations:**
    -   Childbirth Organization: www.childbirth.org/
    -   Childbirth and Postpartum Professional Association: www.cappa.net
    -   Lamaze International: www.lamaze.com/

Child Psychiatric Nurse

1. **Basic description** — A nurse who works with children and adolescents with psychiatric problems. Focuses on the entire continuum between health and illness. The nurse's role is aimed at promotion and prevention, early intervention and treatment of children with severe mental illness. The child psychiatric nurse practices in a variety of settings such as clinics, schools, community agencies, psychiatric hospitals, day treatment facilities, and public health departments.

    Generalist activities of a child psychiatric nurse include: teaching parents with emotionally disturbed or mentally retarded children or adolescents; participation as a member of a health care delivery team and participation in research activities related to the field of child and adolescent psychiatric nursing.

    Advanced practice activities include: consultant to other professional and nonprofessional groups; independent practice psychotherapy; educating other professionals, administrators, and researchers.

2. **Educational requirements** — RN preparation for generalists, with certification in psychiatric/mental health nursing. Advanced practice certification is available for family psychiatric/mental health nurse practitioners and clinical specialists in child and adolescent psychiatric/mental health nursing.

3. **Core competencies/skills needed:**
   - Ability to meet the child at his or her developmental level
   - Facilitate coordination and collaboration among agencies delivering care to children
   - Provide services to children and their families
   - Flexible, sensitive

4. **Compensation**—Varies with place of employment and geographic location.

5. **Employment outlook**—High

6. **Related Web sites and professional organizations:**
   - American Psychiatric Nurses Association: www.apna.org
   - Association of Child and Adolescent Psychiatric Nurses (ACAPN) Association:
     www.ispn-psych.org/html/acapn.html
   - American Nurses Credentialing Center:
     http://www.nursingworld.org/ancc/index.htm

Clinical Nurse Specialist

1. **Basic description**—The clinical nurse specialist coordinates activities regarding patient care on a specific unit within the hospital. This is an advanced practice role and requires a MSN degree. The setting is usually inpatient hospital and intense. Clinical nurse specialists assist the multidisciplinary team from admission to discharge, answer and refer questions the family might have, health teaching, support/counseling, assist in developing protocols for managing care of the client, serve as a resource person to staff nurses and other health team members, collect data and investigate trends for the program, that is, heart surgery, facilitate discharge preparation for a smooth transmission to home, and coordinate follow-up visits for the patient.

2. **Educational requirements** — RN preparation; MSN degree required. Most settings require 5 years of acute care experience.

3. **Core competencies/skills needed:**
   - Must have self-confidence and strong leadership skills
   - Excellent communication
   - Understand organizational structure
   - Technical competency involving use of complex equipment
   - Teaching skills
   - Clinical competency
   - Ability to work with interdisciplinary teams
   - Skills in staff evaluation

4. **Compensation** — Varies with place of employment and geographic location; range is $60,000 to $90,000.

5. **Employment outlook** — Moderate

6. **Related Web sites and nursing organizations:**
   - National Association of Clinical Nurse Specialists (NACNS): www.nacns.org
   - American Board of Nursing Specialties (ABNS): www.nursingcertification.org
   - American Nurses Credentialing Center: www.nursingworld.org/ancc/index.htm

Consultant

1. **Basic description** — A consultant is one who gives advice or provides specialized services on an hourly or contractual basis; nurse consultants can provide advice and/or services in a wide range of areas, such as research development, clinical areas of expertise (diabetes, cardiovascular disease), curriculum development, staffing of health care institutions, and so forth. A consultant might work or practice in virtually any and all aspects of

the health care industry, including private practice. Health care in general, and nursing in particular provide a wide range of opportunities for consultants. Services can be provided as part of a group effort or by an individual with a specific area of expertise.

2. **Educational requirements**—RN preparation; often additional education is required in the consultant's area of expertise. For example, research consultants would have PhD degrees; clinical consultants would have graduate degrees in their clinical area of specialization.

3. **Core competencies/skills needed:**
    *   Requires independent functioning and team skills, with a clear focus on results that are contracted for by the client
    *   Entrepreneurial skills
    *   Communication skills
    *   Organizational skills
    *   Writing ability
    *   Leadership skills
    *   Project management skills

4. **Compensation**—Varies with the client; can range as high as consultants in other professions.

5. **Employment outlook**—High

6. **Related Web site and professional organization:**
    *   National Nurses in Business Association: www.nnba.net

---

Correctional Facility Nurse

1. **Basic description**—The nurse who works in a correctional facility provides health care for all inmates. This includes case management, responding to episodes of acute illness, managing emergency calls, psychiatric evaluations, and assessment of new

inmates. Types of patients are those with health problems related to chronic illness, AIDS, substance abuse, renal failure/dialysis, respiratory diseases, and terminal cancer.

2. **Educational requirements**—RN preparation. Positions are entry level and orientation and assignment to a preceptor is required in most correctional facilities.

3. **Core competencies/skills needed**—The nurse who works in a correctional facility needs strong basic nursing skills, including
   - The ability to function to function independently
   - The ability to respond to emergency situations
   - Knowledge of mental health issues
   - Health promotion and disease prevention skills
   - Strong assessment skills

4. **Compensation**—Varies with geographic location, type, and size of correctional facility.

5. **Employment outlook**—High

6. **Related Web site and professional organization:**
   - Official Home of Corrections: www.corrections.com

Critical Care Nurse

1. **Basic description**—A critical care nurse cares for a small number of patients, usually between one and three, who are critically ill. The nurse has a great deal of one-on-one contact with the patient and is often the main source of contact for the family members. A critical care nurse is responsible for constant monitoring of the patient's condition, as well as recognition of any subtle changes. These nurses use a large amount of technology within their practice and function as integral members of the multidisciplinary health care team. Critical care nurses must

possess the ability to collaborate with other members of the health care team such as physicians, case managers, therapists, and especially other nurses. They are responsible for all care given to the patient, from bed baths to medication administration to tracheotomy and other ventilator care, as well as constant monitoring of the patient for any alterations in their status. Responsibilities include monitoring, assessment, vital sign monitoring, ventilatory management, medication administration, IV insertion and infusion, caring for central lines, Swan-Ganz catheters, and maintaining a running record of the patient's status. Must be prepared at all times to perform CPR and other lifesaving techniques.

2. **Educational requirements**—RN preparation, ACLS certification are required. BSN and CCRN preferred, may be required, depending on the institution. Most institutions require at least 1 to 2 years of medical/surgical experience, although some hospitals are offering extended preceptorships to selected new graduates. Previous critical care experience is desired. In addition to prior experience, many institutions require nurses to pass a critical care course, usually offered in the hospital, and complete 4 to 6 weeks of orientation to the unit.

3. **Core competencies/skills needed:**
   - Excellent assessment skills; ability to detect very subtle changes in a patient's condition
   - Strong organizational skills; ability to prioritize
   - Communication skills and patient and family education skills
   - Strong knowledge of anatomy and physiology, medications and their actions, interactions, side effects, and calculations
   - Maturity and ability to handle end of life issues such as when to cease life prolonging interventions or organ donation decisions
   - An affinity for technology

4. **Compensation**—Varies with place of employment and geographic location.

5. **Employment outlook**—High

6. **Related Web site and professional organization:**
   - American Association of Critical-Care Nurses (AACN): www.aacn.org

Cruise Ship/Resort Nurse

1. **Basic description**—Cruise ship/resort nurses work on ships or at resorts to provide emergency and general care to passengers/vacationers, should it be required. These nurses also serve as part of the occupational health team for crew members who live on the ship for 6 to 8 months at a time, or for the staff at resorts. Responsibilities include providing patient care in the Health Center and dealing with on-site emergencies. This work offers flexibility! Assignments are 3- to 6-month contract positions, living and working with the same people, and meeting people from around the world. Responsibilities include

   • Providing patient care both on a day-to-day basis and in emergency situations
   • Maintaining rapport with guests, physicians, and other crew members
   • Communicating to arrange for workers or guests to receive medical attention
   • Providing discharge instructions for each patient
   • Preparing and maintaining medical records and billing for all patients
   • Complying with resort and maritime rules, regulations, and procedures

2. **Educational requirements**—RN preparation with a minimum of 2 years of recent hospital experience required. Experience with cardiac care, trauma, and internal medicine is desirable.

3. **Core competencies/skills needed:**

   • Must possess excellent interpersonal skills, enjoy traveling, and be flexible
   • Excellent communication skills

- Strong health assessment skills
- Possess a valid passport
- Able to advise patients with colds, headaches, or other minor illnesses

4. **Compensation**—Salaries range from $28,000 to $35,000, depending on the location or the cruise line.

5. **Employment outlook**—Moderate

6. **Related Web sites and professional organizations:**
   - Cruise Line Employment:
     www.cruiselinejob.com/medical.htm
   - Nursing Spectrum Career Fitness Online; *Cruising to a New Opportunity*, by Pat Clutter, RN, MEd, CEN:
     http://nsweb.nursingspectrum.com/cfforms/cruising.cfm

Diabetes Educator

1. **Basic description**—The diabetic educator works with diabetic patients to teach them about diabetes and how to live a healthy life with this very common health problem. Most diabetic educators work in clinics or physician offices and manage the care of the clients with this disease. The diabetic nurse educator establishes long-time commitments and knows patients very well. Responsibilities include instruction on foot and skin care, and appropriate diet; monitoring of blood glucose; administration of insulin; knowledge of hypoglycemia and hyperglycemia; and keeping up with the newest techniques and interventions available

2. **Educational requirements**—The care of diabetic patients is very complex and requires a minimum of a BSN and special certification as a diabetic educator. Increasingly, MSN preparation is required.

3. **Core competencies/skills needed**—Extensive expertise and knowledge about the care of diabetic patients, patient education skills, and interpersonal skills.
4. **Compensation**—The salary range is from $40,000 to $60,000, depending on education and experience.
5. **Employment outlook**—Moderate
6. **Related Web site and nursing organization:**
   • American Association of Diabetes Educators (AADE): www.aadenet.org

Disaster/Bioterrorism Nurse

1. **Basic description**—The disaster/bioterrorism nurse works in disaster areas that are the result of a bioterrorist attack or in situations caused by natural disaster, war, or poverty. Red Cross nurses are often part of the network that provides assistance during times of disaster or conflict. The nature of the work will vary depending on the course of the disaster or conflict.
2. **Educational requirements**—RN preparation. Red Cross nurses must have special training and 20 hours of volunteer or paid service before being assigned to a disaster situation.
3. **Core competencies/skills needed:**
   • Emergency room or critical care experience
   • Experience with local disaster action teams
   • Management skills
   • Ability to meet the needs of people in crisis and high stress situations
   • Knowledge of disaster preparedness and basic first aid
4. **Compensation**—Varies with place of employment and geographic location. No compensation if volunteer effort.

5. **Employment outlook**—Moderate to high
6. **Related Web sites and professional organizations:**
   - American Red Cross: www.redcross.org
   - American Nurses Association: Bioterrorism and Disaster Response: www.nursingworld.org/news/disaster/

Editor

1. **Basic description**—Nurse who works in any area of scientific or professional editing including proofreading and copyediting of technical material. This material may be used in research, biomedical research, education, training, sales and marketing, and other medical mediums and communication forms. This specialty combines editing and writing skills with medical knowledge, and there are numerous opportunities for freelance work that can be done from home with flexible hours. Sometimes the work can be isolating and the data can be very technical, detail oriented, tedious, and voluminous; however, the work varies depending on content being edited. Opportunities exist to work for medical marketing/communications companies, pharmaceutical companies, medical and general interest publications, medical education companies, and professional organizations.

2. **Educational requirements**—RN preparation; BSN or higher often required.

3. **Core competencies/skills needed:**
   - Excellent writing skills
   - Good command of the English language
   - Attention to detail
   - Strong organizational and analytical skills
   - Ability to work alone
   - Ability to meet deadlines

- Excellent computer skills
- Health care–related knowledge

4. **Compensation**—Varies with the place of employment
5. **Employment outlook**—High
6. **Related Web sites and professional organizations:**
   - Registered Nurse Experts, Inc.: www.rnexperts.com
   - Tips to get published: www.medi-smart.com/authors.htm
   - American Medical Writers Association: www.amwa.org

Educator in Academia

1. **Basic description**—College and university faculty who teach and advise students in basic and graduate degree programs in nursing are nurse educators or academic nurses. Faculty may give lectures to several hundred students in large halls, lead small seminars, or supervise students in laboratories. They prepare lectures, exercises, and laboratory experiments; grade exams and papers; and advise and work with students individually. In universities, they also supervise graduate students' teaching and research. Faculty members are expected to keep up with developments in their field by reading current literature and participating in professional conferences. Faculty members consult with government, business, nonprofit, and community organizations. They also do their own research to expand knowledge in their field. They perform experiments; collect and analyze data; and publish their research results in professional journals, books, and electronic media. Most faculty members serve on academic or administrative committees that deal with the policies of their institution, departmental matters, academic issues, curricula, budgets, equipment purchases, and hiring. Some work with student and community organizations. Department chairpersons

are faculty members who usually teach some courses but have heavier administrative responsibilities. Clinical faculty members provide clinical supervision of students.

2. **Educational requirements**—Varies with level of position; college faculty and deans usually need a doctorate (PhD, EdD, DNSc, ND); these individuals serve as the top administrative officer of the academic unit for full-time, tenure-track positions in 4-year colleges and universities; instructors and clinical faculty most often have educational preparation at the master's degree level.

3. **Core competencies/skills needed:**
   - Strong interpersonal and communication skills
   - Motivational and mentoring skills
   - Knowledge of teaching/learning and/or management principles and practices
   - Ability to make sound decisions and to organize and coordinate work efficiently
   - Time management skills; ability to work independently and manage a large number of diverse projects
   - Research and publication skills, especially for faculty at professorial ranks in colleges and universities
   - Ability to manage a flexible schedule; faculty must be present for classes, usually 12 to 16 hours per week, and for faculty and committee meetings. Most faculty establish regular office hours for student consultations, usually 3 to 6 hours per week. Otherwise, faculty are free to decide when and where they will work, and how much time to devote to course preparation, grading, study, research, graduate student supervision, and other activities.

4. **Compensation**—Earnings for college faculty vary according to rank and type of institution, geographic location, and field of specialization. Salaries for full-time faculty average $58,000, with a range of $35,000 for lecturers/instructors to $90,000 for professors. In addition to typical benefits, most college and university faculty enjoy some unique benefits, including access to campus facilities, tuition waivers for dependents, housing and travel allowances, and paid sabbatical leaves.

5. **Employment outlook**—High. There is a serious and growing shortage of nurse faculty.
6. **Related Web sites and professional organizations:**
    *   National League for Nursing (NLN): www.nln.org
    *   American Association of Colleges of Nursing (AACN): www.aacn.nche.edu

---

Emergency Room Nurse

1. **Basic description**—Emergency department (ED) or emergency room (ER) nurses specialize in trauma and critical care, working in environments that are specially equipped to manage emergency care in life-threatening circumstances. ED nurses are often on the front line of health care as many persons use the emergency room as their primary source of care.
2. **Educational requirements**—RN preparation with 1 to 3 years of acute care experience. Although not required by all emergency rooms, ED nurses are usually trained in advanced cardiac support and pediatric advanced life support. Certification is available from the Board of Certification for Emergency Nursing.
3. **Core competencies/skills needed:**
    *   Organization skills
    *   Ability to triage patients
    *   Mental ability to deal with death and dying
    *   Ability to take medical histories and make accurate assessments quickly
    *   Ability to manage mass casualty situations
    *   Technical proficiency with health care equipment
    *   Ability to function in high-stress situations
4. **Compensation**—Varies with place of employment and geographic location.

5. **Employment outlook**—High
6. **Related Web sites and professional organizations:**
   - Emergency Nurses Association: www.ena.org
   - Willy's Emergency Nursing Web:
     www.virtualnurse.com/er/er.html

Entrepreneur

1. **Basic description**—Nurse who starts his/her own business, assuming all risk and responsibility. These entrepreneurs may work in any aspect of the health care/medical industry. Examples of settings include both independent practice or corporations and industry.
2. **Educational requirements**—RN license required. BSN and MSN desired. Degree in business is helpful.
3. **Core competencies/skills needed:**
   - Must possess desire to have own business and/or practice independently
   - Excellent communication skills
   - Independent individual who is flexible, autonomous, and has creative freedom
   - Self-motivated, ambitious, determined, and self-confident
   - Willing to take risks and make important decisions
4. **Compensation**—Salary is self-generated; nurse entrepreneurs are responsible for their own health care and other benefits.
5. **Employment outlook**—High
6. **Related Web sites and professional organizations:**
   - National Nurses in Business Association (NNBA):
     www.nnba.net
   - U.S. Small Business Administration: www.sba.gov

Epidemiology Nurse

1. **Basic description**—A nurse epidemiologist investigates trends in groups or aggregates and studies the occurrence of diseases and injuries. The information is gathered from census data, vital statistics, and reportable disease records. Nurse epidemiologists identify people or populations at high risk; monitor the progress of diseases; specify areas of health care need; determine priorities, size, and scope of programs; and evaluate their impact. They generally do not provide direct patient care, but serve as a resource and plan educational programs. They also publish results of studies and statistical analysis of morbidity and mortality. Examples of practice settings are the Centers for Disease Control and Prevention (CDC) in Atlanta, Georgia, public health departments, and governmental agencies.

2. **Educational requirements**—Masters degree in Public Health or Community Health Nursing. PhD preferred.

3. **Core competencies/skills needed:**
   - Must possess mathematical and analytical ability
   - Have knowledge of both infectious and noninfectious diseases
   - Desire to improve the health and well-being of populations
   - Ability to identify populations at risk
   - Knowledge of health policy
   - Plan programs and health services

4. **Compensation**—Varies with place of employment and geographic location.

5. **Employment outlook**—High

6. **Related Web sites and professional organizations:**
   - Centers for Disease Control and Prevention: www.cdc.gov
   - Association for Professionals in Infection Control and Epidemiology, Inc. (APIC): www.apic.org

Ethicist

1. **Basic description**—An ethicist is a nurse who knows about legal/moral/ethical issues and provides services for patients and families. The nurse ethicist may work with an ethics team to develop a detailed investigative plan to answer questions raised by an ethics violation allegation or resolve ethical dilemmas. Opportunities exist to work in hospitals, nursing homes, hospices, and outpatient settings.

2. **Educational requirements**—RN preparation; MSN or graduate degree in bioethics or related field.

3. **Core competencies/skills needed:**
   - Requires technical training and previous experience with investigations
   - Excellent communication skills
   - Involves conducting and documenting investigations
   - May include interviewing and/or reviewing documents that may pertain to the allegations
   - Knowledge of ethical and legal issues surrounding end-of-life care
   - Knowledge of compliance-related concepts, policies, and procedures
   - Knowledge of all faiths and beliefs
   - Must be able to work well with others to draw conclusions based on allegations
   - Expertise in pain management and issues of loss and grief are helpful

4. **Compensation**—Varies with place of employment and geographic location.

5. **Employment outlook**—Moderate

6. **Related Web sites and professional organizations:**
   - Nursing Ethics Network: www.nusingethicsnetwork.org/
   - Nursing World Ethics: www.nusingworld.org/ethics/
   - Hospice Foundation of America: www.hospicefoundation.org/

Family Nurse Practitioner

1. **Basic description**—Family nurse practitioners (FNPs) are advanced practice nurses who specialize in providing health promotion and care to patients in primary care settings. The FNP provides primary screenings and focuses on health promotion and disease prevention across the life span. Family nurse practitioners have many of the same duties as acute care practitioners, but typically do not work with patients who are critically ill. Family nurse practitioners perform physical examinations, order diagnostic tests, establish diagnoses, prescribe medications, and educate patient and family members regarding health and illness conditions and treatment plans. Examples of settings in which a FNP might practice are physicians' offices, health care clinics, private practice, hospitals, long-term care facilities, public health departments, and occupational health settings.

2. **Educational requirements**—MSN with advanced practice certification as a Family Nurse Practitioner (FNP). Programs are generally 2 years in length combining clinical and didactic work.

3. **Core competencies/skills needed:**
   - Ability to perform physical exams
   - Ability to assess accurately when doing screenings and diagnostic tests; knowledge of normal ranges and abnormal findings
   - Strong communication skills

- Teaching ability and interest
- Ability to work with interdisciplinary teams as well as functioning independently
- Knowledge of acute and chronic conditions
- Excellent judgment in knowing when to make a referral
- Prescribing of medications

4. **Compensation**—Salaries vary according to place of employment and geographic location.

5. **Employment outlook**—Moderate

6. **Related Web sites and professional organizations:**
   - American Academy of Nurse Practitioners (AANP): www.aanp.org
   - American College of Nurse Practitioners (ACNP): www.nurse.org/acnp

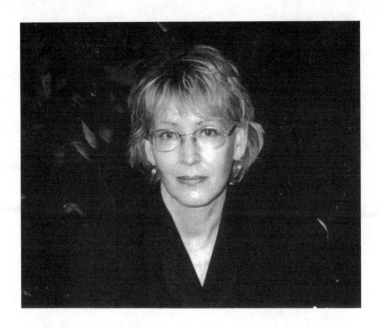

Nancy Hamlin, Family Nurse Practitioner.

An Interview with
Nancy Hamlin,
Family Nurse Practitioner

What is your educational background in nursing (and other areas) and what formal credentials do you hold?

I have a BS degree in nursing from Vanderbilt University and an MS in nursing from Tennessee State University. I am a Family Nurse Practitioner certified by ANCC.

How did you first become interested in your current career?

I started nursing school because of a federally funded program for LPN students and I saw it as a way to support myself financially. A few years later, I obtained a 2-year degree in nursing. Several years later I went back for a BSN, then an MSN (FNP). I am now working on a clinical doctorate at Case Western Reserve University. I am a nationally certified FNP through ANCC. I continued my education because it brought me more job security, money, and autonomy.

What are the most rewarding aspects of your career?

I enjoy helping solve health problems for people. I especially enjoy the area of education and counseling. I like to teach graduate students in the clinical area. I feel that I am contributing to the overall health of the community by providing my services.

Describe a typical workday in your current job.

I currently work in a walk-in clinic that is open 12 hours Monday through Friday and 8 hours on the weekends. The pace can be fast and I usually see at least 4 patients an hour. The type of patient that we see is diverse—everything from upper respiratory infections and broken bones to patients who are having chest pains. Sometimes we need to send patients to the ER and we make a lot of follow-up referrals to specialists. Typically there are no scheduled breaks.

What advice would you give to someone contemplating the same career path in nursing?

Try to get career counseling early and complete your education in an organized fashion. Seek out a mentor. Try to project which areas of nursing will be growing so that if you pursue that area you will likely be employed. Be flexible and find a niche or area you can enjoy and also provide a needed service. Continue looking for opportunities for more education and growth.

How do you balance career and other aspects of your life?

I lead a busy life with a husband and two teens, and I work full-time. I think one must be organized; then you can find the time for the things that are important.

Do you have any other advice for other nurses who might want to pursue this type of nursing career?

Nursing has always been rewarding for me. An advanced degree has given me more independence and more opportunity to be exposed to and learn new things. I think that focusing on service to other people brings satisfaction and happiness. I think the role of the advanced practice nurse is unique and to enjoy this career you must see yourself as a valuable part of the health care team.

Flight Nurse/Critical Care Transport

1. **Basic description**—A flight nurse is a highly trained and experienced critical care registered nurse. The flight nurse works with a flight crew most likely consisting of the flight nurse/paramedic, flight respiratory therapist/EMT-1, and a pilot to transport patients to, from, and between hospital facilities. Flight nurses work in intensive care units, emergency rooms, ambulance companies, and emergency transport facilities.

2. **Educational requirements**—BSN prepared RN. Must hold current certification as a Certified Flight RN, Certified Emergency Nurse, or Certified Critical Care Nurse and be certified as a Paramedic. Advanced Cardiac Life Support and Pediatric Advanced Life Support, Neonatal Advanced Life Support, completion of a trauma nurse core curriculum, and completion of a flight nurse advanced trauma course are needed. Usually requires a minimum of 2 to 3 years of critical care nursing experience. Rigorous ongoing continuing education is necessary to support the extensive knowledge and skills that are expected for flight nurses.

3. **Core competencies/skills needed:**
   - Experience in multisystem trauma, neonates, pediatrics, severe burns, acute medical, high-risk obstetrics, and cardiac patients
   - Prepared to utilize endotracheal intubations, use of chemical paralytic agents, and placement of central venous access via the femoral or subclavian route, surgical airways, pericardiocentesis, needle thoracostomy, and intraosseous access

- Assume the responsibility of sharing knowledge about emergency care systems with other members of the health care team, patients, their significant others, and the community
- Involved in research that directly relates to improved patient care in the air medical transport industry, and/or improves the professional standards of practice that promote the flight nurse as a professional
- Responsible for direct patient care during transport, which may include monitoring, medication administration, assessment, IV infusion, ventilatory/airway management, charting, and communication with other health care providers
- Provide the rapid assessment, diagnosis, and treatment of critically injured or ill patients of all ages from the scene of an accident or from referring facilities

4. **Compensation**—Varies with place of employment and geographic location.

5. **Employment outlook**—Moderate

6. **Related Web site and professional organization:**
   - Air and Surface Transport Nurses Association: www.astna.org

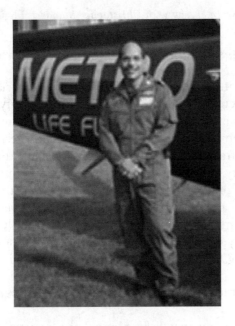

Christopher Manacci, Flight Nurse Specialist.

An Interview with Christopher Manacci, Flight Nurse Specialist

What is your educational background and preparation?

I attended Ursuline College and Lorain County Community College for my undergraduate education in nursing. I then received a master's degree in nursing from Case Western Reserve University in the acute care nurse practitioner program. I am board certified in Critical Care (CCRN), board certified in Flight Nursing (CFRN), and certified as a Trauma Nurse Specialist in the State of Illinois, Department of Public Health.

How did you first become interested in your current career?

I first became interested in flight nursing (a new specialty at the time) while I was practicing in the ICU at a large community-based hospital. I enjoyed the complexity of the ICU patient population, but desired to practice in an environment that required more acute intervention and stabilization. I trained as a Trauma Nurse Specialist then transitioned to the emergency department of an urban level one-trauma center. After several years of practice, I missed the level of sophistication and detail the ICU patient population presented to my practice. Flight Nursing combines the sophistication of an intensive care unit with the urgency of an emergency department. It seemed like the "best of both worlds" as I was looking to increase my level of practice and capability.

What are the most rewarding aspects of your career?

There is no question that I am granted the greatest privilege of any professional within or outside the health profession. On a daily basis I am given the privilege to care for the most critical of patients in their greatest time of need. My practice spans all age groups in every clinical subspecialty. I am able to be the human interface of the most technologically advanced interventions, while encouraging physiological survival. Also, I serve as a link to individuals, families, and communities who may otherwise not benefit from the access to specialty care centers. Nurses have always been the clinician of choice since the inception of air medical services owing to their unique academic preparation in the physical, psychological, and social sciences, armed with clinical knowledge and critical thinking skills inherent to our profession. Today with the health care system under siege, I am proud to be a part of "what is right" about the health care system. I believe it was the French philosopher Voltaire who said "Men [women] who save lives partake in divinity, whereas saving a life is almost as noble as creating one." It is nurses that have the greatest opportunity to achieve this.

Describe a typical workday in your current job.

On any given "typical" day the only certainty is uncertainty. I report for duty at 0700 hours and receive report from the off-going flight nurse specialist including accounting of narcotics stored. Then I prepare for and complete my routine duties of the shift, such as checking expiration dates and temperature range of stored blood used for missions. I am scheduled for 12 or 24 hours. First I check the equipment and supplies aboard the S-76 aircraft (helicopter). This is essential as I do not have the luxury of calling CSR (Central Supply Room) or pharmacy for missing items as the need may arise when I am caring for a patient on a freeway, in a cornfield, or at 1,500 feet while moving 180 mph. We provide routine nursing care, such as assessment, planning, intervention, and evaluation, as well as advanced procedures of airway management, central line placement, tube thoracostomy, and emergent surgical interventions. Preplanning for the unknown is the common denominator in flight nursing practice. There is no way to anticipate what type of mission awaits you, but a mission of some type is certain. On any given day you may care for an adult with a life-threatening medical condition or a young child critically injured by a car crash, or both. You may be called for a high-risk obstetrical patient or a premature infant born with a congenital heart defect. Nonetheless, you will be called and must be prepared. I have completed as many as 7 missions in a 12-hour shift. As a program with three online helicopters we have completed as many as 26 missions in a 24-hour period.

What advice would you give to someone contemplating the same career path in nursing?

The advice I would give someone contemplating the same career path is that every specialty in nursing provides you with unique opportunities, but flight nursing provides you with all of them. It is necessary to have a strong clinical background in critical care nursing and a strong understanding of pathophysiology, pharmacology, and clinical management of a variety of disease processes. It is essential that you enjoy caring for critically ill and injured patients in an unstructured environment. The best preparation is a clinically proficient individual who is formally trained in the notions of autonomous and collaborative practice. I believe it is helpful if you have completed research related to the care of individuals and have the ability to evaluate and implement current therapeutic interventions. The most important asset is the desire to make a difference and the passion to alter the outcome of those entrusted to your care.

How do you balance career and other aspects of your life?

Balance is always an interesting question. Flight nursing practice is of extremes, so balance is often achieved by participating in activities or events that compensate for that particular day or week. For instance, if I participate in a particularly socially difficult mission, I may choose to have quiet time with my family. Although we participate in many triumphs, there is a significant amount of tragedy. Flight nurses do not merely observe tragic events, they participate in them, so a strong sense of who you are is helpful. Since there is not much control over the type or consistency of missions, it is necessary to have consistency in your personal life. Eating well, resting, and a regular workout routine are helpful.

Do you have any other advice for other nurses who might want to pursue this type of nursing career?

Gain as much education and knowledge as early in your career as possible, do not jump from unit to unit, rather understand the practice expectations in the process of caring for patients. This, coupled with clinical expertise and skill proficiencies, will provide you with the ability to be a strong candidate for a flight nursing position. More important, it will provide you with the tools to care for your patients in any setting.

Thank you for undertaking this important work and for allowing me to participate. I truly believe that nursing is important and so should the rest of the world.

Forensic Nurse

1. **Basic description**—Forensic nurses combine clinical nursing practice in conjunction with knowledge of law enforcement. They provide care to victims and are involved in the investigation of sexual assault, elder and spousal abuse, and unexplained or accidental death. Forensic nursing is high stress because of the nature of the work, and it requires a broad understanding of social, environmental, and psychological influences on behavior. The environments in which forensic nurses work are varied. They work in such settings as correctional institutions, psychiatric facilities, acute care settings, coroner and medical examiners' offices, and for insurance companies.

2. **Educational requirements**—RN preparation; BSN required and often graduate preparation. Certification from SANE may also be needed for some practice settings.

3. **Core competencies/skills needed:**
    *   Must be able to work in diverse conditions and deal with emotionally charged issues.
    *   Ability to combine nursing knowledge with investigative and counseling skills
    *   Ability to collaborate with experts in other disciplines
    *   Be an advocate for victims
    *   Coordinate programs in collaboration with medical and law enforcement
    *   Be able to deal with death and dying

4. **Compensation**—Varies according to place of employment and geographic location.

5. **Employment outlook**—Moderate

6. **Related Web site and professional organization:**
    *   Forensic Nursing Services (FNS): www.forensicnursing.org

Fraud and Abuse Investigator

1. **Basic description** — A fraud and abuse investigator investigates health care fraud and abuse charges using such techniques as information technology and statistics to identify outlier practice behaviors. They are employed by government agencies investigating abuse or fraud, or by independent consulting groups who perform this service through contacts with government agencies. This allows investigators to recognize and look more closely at providers who are practicing in an unusual manner. Investigations are often aggressive and involve working with the FBI and U.S. States Attorneys to obtain justice. Cases are also reported to local medical and professional boards. The most common types of fraud and abuse are upcoding (for example, a practitioner billing for a 60-minute office visit when it was only a 20-minute visit); unbundling (for example, usually dealing with CPT coding, like a blood test being billed under a combined code, then one or more tests from that composite test gets billed individually); charging for services not rendered; and performing unnecessary procedures or tests.

2. **Educational requirements** — RN preparation and an undergraduate degree are the baseline on which to add additional skills, certifications, and expertise. Graduate degree in business is desired.

3. **Core competencies/skills needed:**
    *   Computer literacy. Cases are often complex with myriad databases requiring an understanding of information technology
    *   A broad background in nursing with up-to-date clinical knowledge
    *   Experience and understanding of the health care system

- Law-related areas of study are valuable, as is an in-depth understanding of managed care, risk management, and contracts
- Understanding of annual reports and budgets
- An understanding of statistics is important because current investigative technique is often computer generated and driven and involves the use of statistics
- Recognition that the cost of fraud is paid by everyone and that health care dollars are finite
- An understanding that money spent on dishonest reimbursement reduces the amount of money available for preventative and other appropriate care

4. **Compensation**—Varies with place of employment and geographic location.

5. **Employment outlook**—High

6. **Related Web site and professional organization:**
   - EDS: Electronic Data Systems
   - http://www.eds.com/health_care/medicaid/hc_medicaid_white_paper_dec.shtml

Gastroenterology Nurse

1. **Basic description**—Gastroenterology nursing is a specialty practice area in which nurses provide care to patients with known or suspected gastrointestinal problems and are undergoing diagnostic or therapeutic treatment and/or procedures. This area of nursing has expanded because of increased technology and new screening procedures. Practice environments are usually available in endoscopy departments in hospitals, clinics, or physicians' offices, as well as ambulatory outpatient endoscopy facilities.

2. **Educational requirements**—RN preparation. National certification in the specialty is available through the Certifying Board of Gastroenterology Nurses. This board sets the requirements for obtaining and maintaining certification. Certified Registered Nurses earn the credential Certified Gastroenterology Registered Nurse (CGRN). Generally nurses have experience in medical-surgical nursing prior to electing to specialize.

3. **Core competencies/skills needed:**
   - Technical competency
   - Maturity
   - Empathy
   - Knowledge of pathophysiology of gastrointestinal system
   - Physical assessment and screening skills
   - Case management skills

4. **Compensation**—Varies depending on place of employment and the geographic location.

5. **Employment outlook**—Moderate

6. **Related Web sites and professional organizations:**
   - Society of Gastroenterology Nurses and Associates, Inc. (SGNA): www.sgna.org
   - Gastroenterology Nursing: www.gastroenterologynursing.com
   - Certifying Board of Gastroenterology Nurses and Associates, Inc. (CBGNA): www.cbgna.org/

Genetics Counselor

1. **Basic description**—Genetic counselors are nurses or health professionals with specialized graduate degrees and experience in the areas of genetics and counseling. Most enter the field from a variety of disciplines, including biology, genetics, nursing,

psychology, public health, and social work. Genetic counselors frequently speak to clients about complex scientific and emotional topics. They work as members of a health care team providing information and support to families who have members with birth defects or genetic disorders and to families who may be at risk for a variety of inherited conditions. Genetic counselors investigate the problem present in the family, interpret information about the disorder, analyze inheritance patterns and risks of recurrence, review available options with the family, serve as patient advocates, and engage in research activities.

2. **Educational requirements**—Educational requirements for the nurse would be a master's degree or PhD with advanced education in genetics such as that offered through the National Institutes of Health. The American Board of Genetic Counseling certifies genetic counselors and accredits genetic counseling training programs. Certification in genetic counseling is available by the American Board of Genetic Counseling (ABGC). Requirements include documentation of the following: a graduate degree in genetic counseling; clinical experience in an ABGC-approved training site or sites; a log book of 50 supervised cases; and successful completion of both the general and specialty certification examination.

3. **Core competencies/skills needed:**
    *   Knowledge of inherited diseases and the ability to counsel parents and families regarding genetic possibilities
    *   Critical thinking skills
    *   Collaborative team practice skills
    *   Deep sensitivity to patient and family concerns
    *   Listening skills
    *   Maturity

4. **Compensation**—Salary is highly variable.

5. **Employment outlook**—High

6. **Related Web sites and professional organizations:**
    *   National Society of Genetic Counselors, Inc. (NSGC): www.nsgc.org
    *   Online Journal of Genetic Counseling: www.kluweronline.com/issn/1059-7700

- The American Board of Genetic Counseling, Inc. (ABGC): www.faseb.org/genetics/abgc/abgcmenu.htm

Geriatric Nurse Practitioner

1. **Basic description**—Geriatric nurse practitioners (GNPs) provide primary and acute care to older persons. They work in hospitals, nursing homes, clinics, home care agencies, senior citizen centers, and in wellness programs in the community.
2. **Educational requirements**—RN preparation and a graduate degree from a gerontological nurse practitioner program is required.
3. **Core competencies/skills needed:**
   - Skills in development and implementation of treatment plans for chronic illness
   - Ability to provide support, education, and counseling for families
   - Understanding of the special needs of the elderly and the process of aging
   - Skills in coordination of care
4. **Compensation**—Varies with place of employment and geographic location.
5. **Employment outlook**—High
6. **Related Web sites and professional organizations:**
   - National Association of Professional Geriatric Care Managers: www.caremanager.org/
   - National Gerontological Nursing Association: www.ngna.org/
   - American Academy of Nurse Practitioners (AANP): www.aanp.org
   - American College of Nurse Practitioners (ACNP): www.nurse.org/acnp

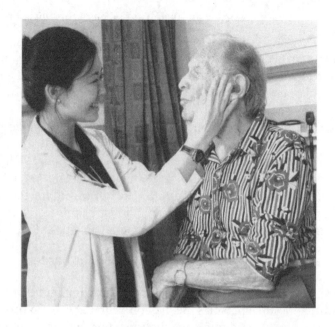

Annie Siu-Lin, Geriatric Nurse Practitioner, with patient.

An Interview with
Annie Siu-Lin,
Geriatric Nurse Practitioner

What is your educational background in nursing (and other areas) and what formal credentials do you hold?

I graduated from the State University of New York (SUNY) at Stony Brook with a BSN degree in 1996. Then I attended New York University Division of Nursing and completed a graduate degree in 1998 to become an Advanced Practice Nurse and Geriatric Nurse Practitioner.

How did you first become interested in your current career?

I first became interested in geriatric nursing when I was doing my summer undergraduate clinical internship at SUNY Stony Brook Hospital. I was assigned to a Geriatric Unit and realized that I was more interested in working with elderly patients than with any other age group or specialty. When working with geriatric patients I frequently came upon misconceptions from other health care workers regarding care and treatment of the elderly. It was also very challenging because there was never a simple and easy solution; there was always a holistic approach to the many problems that elderly patients have. With this I found working with the elderly very challenging and yet felt that I could make a positive change and difference in caring for them. I also wanted to directly make changes with a holistic approach and felt the best way to do this was by becoming a Geriatric Nurse Practitioner.

What are the most rewarding aspects of your career?

The most rewarding aspect of my career is knowing and being able to make a difference in a person's life. Not only am I able to do this directly by seeing patients and doing consultations, but my responsibility also includes implementing best practice protocols and educating all health staff to provide the best quality, compassionate and culturally appropriate care for every senior admitted to the hospital. Knowing that I can improve care for the elderly makes my job as a Geriatric Nurse Practitioner very rewarding.

Describe a typical workday in your current job.

A typical workday as a Geriatric Nurse Practitioner in my current job would be making rounds with nurses and physicians, in addition to seeing patients as a consultant and targeting specific issues such as patients with dementia, delirium, depression, restraint usage, high risk for falls, pressure ulcers, and palliative care issues. While doing rounds and seeing patients I directly educate all clinical staff on best practice protocols for caring for geriatric patients. In addition, I spend time implementing policies and protocols to ensure that best practice protocols are followed through by all health care staff in the hospital.

What advice would you give to someone contemplating the same career path in nursing?

My advice is know what you wish to accomplish and what your ultimate goals are. If your goal is to become a Geriatric Nurse Practitioner, make that a priority so you will always try to accomplish it. In the end it is always rewarding to be able to pursue your goals no matter how difficult it was to get it done.

How do you balance career and other aspects of your life?

Knowing myself, my limitations and strengths, is the best way for me to balance career and other aspects of my life. I prioritize and try to keep myself organized. When the day is over I tell myself there is always a tomorrow for me to accomplish what I wish to do. I take care of myself so I can take care of others to the best of my abilities. I also try to socialize and collaborate with others so I can accomplish my goals by working with other people and not by myself. Completing goals with a team is always better than with one person.

Do you have any other advice for other nurses who might want to pursue this type of nursing career?

My advice for other nurses who are considering pursuing a career as a Geriatric Nurse Practitioner is to make this a priority once you decide to do this. Get as much clinical experience as you can and keep yourself updated with the newest research. Attend geriatric conferences, join geriatric organizations, and get to know other people who are in the same specialty so you never feel you are alone.

Health Coach

1. **Basic description**—Health coaches are primarily RNs, but also respiratory therapists and dieticians, who work with patients around the clock offering services totally by telephone. They listen with practiced ears and offer support possible from years of clinical experience. They provide state-of-the-art health information from some of the world's top medical experts. They provide a calming voice when a patient is having a crisis or is in pain or indecision, and provide tips on self-care. Health coaches stay in contact with their patients and provide information and support until they begin to feel better and gain confidence. Health coaching has the benefit of time. Coaches have more time with patients to provide them with new tools and more support to help them understand their conditions better and navigate their way through the health care system. Patients will sometimes reveal things over the phone that they would not say in person, fostering deep interactions with their health coach. A large part of health coaching is encouraging patients to become actively involved in their own health and to work with their health care providers in making critical health decisions. Patients are also encouraged to manage their health conditions in ways that reflect the patients' personal values and preferences. Health coaches generally work for independent companies; they also may be independent consultants.

2. **Educational requirements**—RN preparation.

3. **Core competencies/skills needed:**
   - Excellent listening and interpersonal skills based on the fact that all services are telephone based
   - Extensive clinical knowledge

- Knowledge of health promotion, illness prevention, and treatment
- Counseling skills

4. **Compensation**—Varies with place of employment and geographic location.

5. **Employment outlook**—Moderate

6. **Related Web sites and professional organizations:**
   - Health Coach Training Programs and Certification: www.worldhealthandhealing.com/
   - WebMD: www.webmd.com

Health Policy Analyst/Lobbyist

1. **Basic description**—Nurse lobbyists lobby for issues, particularly those related to health care legislation or health policy. A health policy analyst collects data and conducts background research, synthesizes research findings, and reports this information in verbal or written formats, usually on a particular project that serves the client's needs. Because of the analyst's knowledge of health and health care, the data and background documents are framed to convey information about the broad determinants of health and the impact of the data on policy change. A successful lobbyist must perform detailed policy analysis, understand the complex processes of policymaking, establish strong relationships with decision makers, create a trustworthy and approachable reputation, and know the culture of the lawmakers and utilize congruent political strategies. Health policy analysts and lobbyists may be independent consultants or may be employed by professional organizations. Health policy analysts may be employed by government agencies (e.g., state or city health departments).

2. **Educational requirements**—RN preparation; MSN, MPH or equivalent is desired.

3. **Core competencies/skills needed:**
   - Legislative background
   - Analytic skills in public health and health care issues
   - Knowledge of political and legislative processes
   - Appropriate research skills to seek a variety of data sources, and prioritize among the data sources for accuracy and bias
   - Excellent and accurate attention to detail is required in all written and verbal communication
   - Ability to effectively prioritize project tasks and schedules
   - Broad knowledge of key processes related to legislation, regulation, and politics on the local, state, and legislative levels
   - Ability to extract and summarize large amounts of data and evidence to support health policies

4. **Compensation**—Varies with place of employment and geographic location.

5. **Employment outlook**—Moderate

6. **Related Web sites and professional organizations:**
   - State of CT ethics commission lobbyist electronic filing: www.lims.state.CT.us/public/eth4b.asp
   - North Carolina Nurses Association: www.ncnurses.org/leg_info.htm

---

Historian

1. **Basic description**—The nurse historian documents and identifies the dilemmas with which nursing has struggled throughout time. History provides current nurses with the same intellectual and political tools that determined nursing pioneers applied to shape nursing values and beliefs to the social context of their

times. Nursing history includes the study of labor history, gender studies, oral and social history, anthropology, and the social sciences. Such study exposes nursing students, practitioners, faculty, and administrators to the helpfulness of using history to understand the evolution of the profession. It provides a historical perspective to debates on health policy, encourages reflective practice among nursing professionals, and provides the historical legacy of the profession. Nurse historians are most often employed by academic institutions and the historical research is completed as part of their scholarship.

2. **Educational requirements**—PhD is required to do the historical research and to hold a university faculty position as a nurse historian.

3. **Core competencies/skills needed:**
   - Interest in doing historical research and teaching
   - Ability to attend to details
   - Skills in historical research methods

4. **Compensation**—Varies with employment setting and geographic location.

5. **Employment outlook**—Moderate

6. **Related Web sites and professional organizations:**
   - American Association for the History of Nursing, Inc.: www.aahn.org
   - American Nurses Association (ANA) Hall of Fame: www.ana.org/hof/index.htm#about

HIV/AIDS Specialist

1. **Basic description**—Nurse who works primarily with patients inflicted with HIV/AIDS. HIV/AIDS specialists may work in acute care, long-term care facilities, home care, and hospice.

2. **Educational requirements**—RN preparation. Palliative care certification is available, but not always required for job placement; certification by ANAC is available.

3. **Core competencies/skills needed:**
   - Expertise in caring for those who have HIV/AIDS
   - Extensive knowledge of HIV/AIDS disease process
   - Knowledge of death, dying, and grieving process
   - Skills to provide counseling to families of those inflicted with HIV/AIDS
   - Ability to care, manage, and teach those inflicted
   - Assessment skills for pain and pain management techniques
   - Knowledge and understanding of the ethical issues that arise at the end of life

4. **Compensation**—Varies with place of employment and geographical location.

5. **Employment outlook**—High

6. **Related Web sites and professional organizations:**
   - Association of Nurses in AIDS Care: www.anacnet.org
   - World Home Care and Hospice Organization (WHHO): www.whho.org

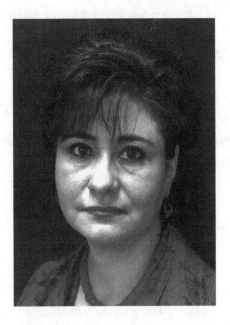

Ingrid Hansen, HIV Specialist Nurse.

An Interview with Ingrid Hansen, HIV Specialist Nurse

What is your educational background in nursing (and other areas) and what formal credentials do you hold?

I received my BSN degree in 1983 from the University of Chile in Valaraiso, Chile. I then became a public health nurse in California and worked in a number of settings in California and Illinois before moving to Texas. I am licensed as a nurse in Illinois, California, and Texas. I am certified as an AIDS nurse, and I am a HIV counselor and a family planning counselor. My current position is as a patient educator for a county health district, assessing the needs of HIV positive pregnant and nonpregnant women.

How did you first become interested in your current career?

At an early age (6 years old), I expressed the desire to be a nurse. I used to play with my dolls pretending that I was giving them injections, or cough syrup. Perhaps because I suffered from asthma from an early age, I was more exposed to doctor's visits and many medications. When I entered nursing school at the age of seventeen, I did not have a doubt in my mind that I was doing the right thing, and now, 25 years later, I still think that it was the best decision that I could ever made.

What are the most rewarding aspects of your career?

One of the most rewarding aspects of my work is knowing that I am touching the lives of others and helping them to change their lives in a positive way. For instance, 2 weeks ago I taught one of my pregnant patients who is illiterate and mentally challenged how to take her antiretroviral therapy, and later on check her viral load which is decreasing in number, which means there is less risk of perinatal transmission.

Describe a typical workday in your current job.

I meet with my patients most of whom are minority women who are HIV positive, during the clinic. Previously I would have participated in a multidisciplinary meeting where I identified the patients' knowledge deficits. I meet with them after they have been seen by the doctor or nurse practitioner, and I give them information based on their needs. Many of these patients speak only Spanish, and some of them are illiterate in both languages. Many times I translate during the doctor's visit, so we make sure the patient understands everything. Sometimes I meet with the patient during the days when we do not have clinic. I count pills with them, to ensure they are adherent to their treatment, and to prevent resistance to the antiretroviral therapy.

What advice would you give to someone contemplating the same career path in nursing?

The field of HIV is very challenging. This disease is extremely dynamic and is changing all the time. If you like to study, to learn new things, you are in the right place. In HIV nursing you will not be bored. What you knew yesterday may not be applicable tomorrow, but at the same time there are many opportunities to learn and grow.

How do you balance career and other aspects of your life?

At times it has been difficult. I have two children, ages 13 and 8, and two beagle dogs. I have been divorced for 2 years. During those difficult times I found the support of my coworkers and supervisor most advantageous. My faith has helped me to obtain balance. Additionally, my career is a source of satisfaction in my life. I feel highly inspired in my work, and I think that is so important in this field. I try to go out during the weekend with my children and have fun. I try not to take my work home and vice versa. As nurses we have to learn to take care of ourselves in order to care for others.

Do you have any other advice for other nurses who might want to pursue this type of nursing career?

Do it from your heart. You can touch so many lives when they are in need or sick. This career is very rewarding but you have to be committed to it. Remember that you have the capacity to touch and transform the lives of others in a positive way. Perhaps you will be the first person who treats that individual with dignity and compassion like a real human being.

Holistic Health Nurse/ Massage Therapist

1. **Basic description**—Holistic nursing involves all aspects of wellness and healing of a holistic nature, with holism defined as the mind, body, spirit connection. Holistic nurses treat the whole person, not just a disease or symptom. Working as a holistic nurse is a chance to be a part of a growing specialty, but because the field is new, some skepticism still exists. Opportunities for employment exist in health care facilities, holistic health and wellness centers, spas and health clubs, private practices, and pain management centers.

2. **Educational requirements**—RN preparation. Certification in holistic nursing is available from the American Holistic Nurses' Certification Corporation (AHNCC).

3. **Core competencies/skills needed:**
   - Interest in and commitment to focus on wellness, healing, and illness prevention from a more spiritual and natural perspective
   - Commitment to a holistic philosophy
   - Knowledge of complementary and alternative therapies
   - Openness to go beyond the conventions of traditional medicine and health care

4. **Compensation**—Varies with place of employment and geographic location.

5. **Employment outlook**—High

6. **Related Web sites and professional organizations:**
   - American Holistic Nurses Association: www.ahna.org

- The National Association of Nurse Massage Therapists: www.npwh.org/
- The RN Reiki Connection: http://member.aol.com/KarunaRN/

Home Health Nurse

1. **Basic description**—A home health nurse provides nursing care and support to individuals and families in their own homes, assisted living facilities, or nursing homes. This care may be provided before or after acute and long-term illness. Home health nurses may be prepared as generalists for care of all patients or may be specialists (e.g., oncology or geriatric nurses). Home health nurses provide direct patient care in contrast to public or community health nurses whose focus is population based.

2. **Educational requirements**—RN preparation.

3. **Core competencies/skills needed:**
   - Ability to function independently at an optimal level
   - Excellent communication and bedside manner with patients and their families
   - The ability to perceive the patient's needs in relation to the home environment
   - The ability to conform and adapt traditional nursing care to the home environment
   - Knowledge of many cultures and openness to work with people from a wide variety of cultures
   - Excellent assessment skills
   - Autonomy and flexibility

4. **Compensation**—Varies with place of employment and geographic location.

5. **Employment outlook**—High

6. **Related Web sites and professional organizations:**
   - National Association for Home Care: www.nahc.org
   - Home Healthcare Nurses Association (HHNA): www.nahc.org/HHNA
   - Visiting Nurse Associations of America: www.vnaa.org

Hospice and Palliative Care Nurse

1. **Basic description**—Hospice/palliative care nurses work with people who have a terminal illness and are predicted to die within 6 months or less. Hospice/palliative care can take place in a hospice facility, but approximately 90% receive care at home or other residential care institutions. Nurses who work with dying patients and their loved ones must be able to manage dealing with death on a daily basis; the stress of the work requires maturity.

2. **Educational requirements**—RN preparation. Usually 1 to 2 years of experience in home care and oncology is recommended before entering this specialty. Certification is available in this specialty (CHPN) through the Board for Certification of Hospice and Palliative Nurses.

3. **Core competencies/skills needed:**
   - Attention to the psychological, spiritual, physical, and social aspects of care as related to the patient's quality of life
   - Skill in using resources found within the home or other residential site to provide end-of-life nursing care
   - Ability to provide stress relief for dying patients and their families
   - Skill in relieving multiple physical symptoms such as pain, dyspnea, fatigue, anorexia, and delirium

- Skill in helping patients deal with emotional symptoms such as depression, anxiety, and fear associated with facing impending death
- Collaboration with other members of the interdisciplinary team to help to relieve patient suffering

4. **Compensation**—Varies with place of employment and geographic location.
5. **Employment outlook**—High
6. **Related Web sites and professional organizations:**
   - Hospice and Palliative Nurses Association (HPNA): www.hpna.org
   - Hospice Association of America: www.hospice-america.org
   - World Home Care and Hospice Organization (WHHO): www.whho.org
   - End of Life Nursing Education Consortium (ELNEC): www.aacn.nche.edu/elnec

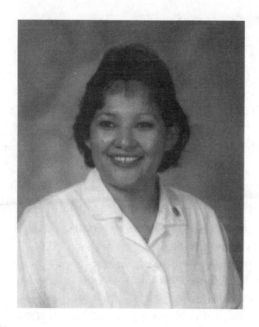

Rose Walls, Palliative Care and Hospice Nurse.

An Interview with Rose Walls, Palliative Care and Hospice Nurse

What is your educational background in nursing (and other areas) and what formal credentials do you hold?

I am a RN with an associate degree in nursing and am certified in hospice and palliative care. Before I became a nurse I was a social worker, but I am not currently licensed in social work. I received a full nursing scholarship from Hospice of Austin; this scholarship program was developed as a means to recruit minorities into nursing. Part of the requirement was a 2-year contract after graduation. My contract was completed in 1998, but I chose to stay because I believe in hospice and palliative care nursing.

How did you first become interested in your current career?

As a young teenager, I was fascinated with the role of a nurse. My cousin was a LVN (licensed vocational nurse) in Michigan, working with a migrant outreach program. She did health assessment and referred people to various community resources to meet their needs for food and other resources. I was her assistant, mainly recording information for her. This later helped me when I was a social worker. It was not until my late 30s that I decided to pursue my first love, nursing.

What are the most rewarding aspects of your career?

The rewards come back to me from patients and families. They open their homes and hearts to me and the rest of the hospice team members. There is no denying their prognosis. Although some of the patients or families appear to remain stoic, there is usually a time in the course of our service in which the situation becomes unavoidable and death becomes real to all of us. It is at this time that we all become a support to one another. I am at awe at the strength of our patients and families as death approaches.

Describe a typical workday in your current job.

I work Monday through Friday. At 7:00 A.M. I listen to voicemail reports regarding situations that may have arisen since the last nurse was there, or since I was there. I determine which patients will be the priority for the day. For example, there may be patients who need increased pain control or other symptom control. Patients who are actively dying (within the next 24 to 48 hours) are given priority. There are times when families are very anxious and nervous and require extra attention to their fears and I would need to provide some immediate support to them. From 8:00 to 10:00 A.M. I usually spend the time on the phone, faxing information related to patients' needs or care to other medical personnel. For example, this time may be spent calling in for medications for patients. I also spend this time contacting patients and families and arranging the times for home visits. I attend meetings and inservice programs at this time. From 10 to 5 each day, I usually visit 4 or 5 patients. Most patient visits are an hour long, but I have been at a home for as long as 4 hours, depending on the patient's needs. At the end of my visits I finish my recordings and paper work. I often will befriend a patient and family within the boundaries of my professional role. For example, I may bring them flowers or sweets when appropriate. Members of the care team have met patients out for lunch and attended weddings or assisted with wedding plans for those who want to get married or renew wedding vows. I also try to attend the funerals of my patients to help provide closure for myself and support to the families. I keep a box full of obituaries, thank-you cards, and other reminders of my care and involvement with patients and families.

What advice would you give to someone contemplating the same career path in nursing?

Those considering nursing must have a love for helping others and a love of nursing. Nursing requires hard work, good judgment, common sense, critical thinking skills, the ability to solve problems, the ability to react quickly in emergency situations, and, at the same time, a sense of calmness and confidence portrayed to families and patients as they are looking to you for guidance and support. Not everyone can do hospice work because of the subject of death. But if you are curious about hospice services, go into hospice care with an open heart to learn about the plan of care (much different from conventional nursing). Our goal is not curative, but palliative. We want to make sure patients and their families are taken care of physically, emotionally, and spiritually. We provide holistic care and it takes all members of the interdisciplinary team for our care to be successful.

How do you balance career and other aspects of your life?

I take care of myself in a holistic manner. Physically, I exercise and try not to skip meals in spite of a busy and hectic schedule. I garden and attend sporting events. Emotionally, I spend quality time with family and spend some time alone, often reading inspiring material. Spiritually, I participate in daily devotions and attend church services regularly. My husband and I lead a food pantry ministry for others; many other nurses participate.

Do you have any other advice for other nurses who might want to pursue this type of nursing career?

The majority of hospice nursing is done in the patients' homes. Families open their homes, their lives, and their hearts to you. At times they treat you as part of their family; you become an important member of their family circle. You will meet people from many different backgrounds. And you will try to be at ease in each setting. I have had patients who are homeless with no caregivers; I also have had patients with paid 24-hour care. Although the settings are different, the care remains the same. This is a challenging career choice in nursing; you will use all of your nursing and personal skills.

Do you have any other advice?

Being a minority in nursing and bilingual (Spanish/English) is more demanding. I am often called upon to help with translations and referrals, and to make visits outside my usual locale as there are not enough bilingual nurses available.

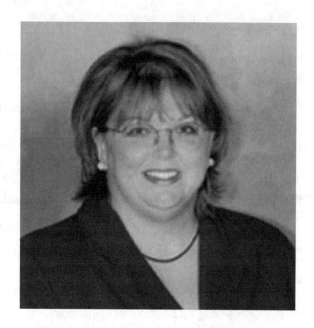

Malene Davis, Hospice Nurse.

An Interview with
Malene Davis,
Hospice Nurse

What is your educational background in nursing (and other areas) and what formal credentials do you hold?

I have a BSN in Nursing, a master's degree in Business Administration, and a master's degree in Nursing. I am certified as a hospice nurse by the Hospice and Palliative Care Nurses Association.

How did you first become interested in your current career?

I became interested in hospice as a nurse who had worked oncology, and then went back to school to pursue an MBA degree. I answered an advertisement that I felt would be an entrance into health care management. I realized after working at hospice that I was fulfilling a ministry, a job God wanted me to do. I was able to work in the community, and that is when I fell in love with my job.

What are the most rewarding aspects of your career?

The most rewarding aspects are working with families and community members. I love teaching them to live life to the fullest—to appreciate each day—to find them help for their needs. I work in a rural, aged part of West Virginia. Resources are limited and when you connect people to benefits they didn't know existed it is wonderful. I love making people feel better—taking the pain away or getting symptoms under control.

Describe a typical workday in your current job.

A typical workday would be to work with staff as they troubleshoot family concerns and decisions facing them. Every family is different and wonderful at the same time, and it takes case-by-case discussion sometimes (chemo, radiation—should I continue, what are the benefits/ pitfalls?). I also help nurses and social workers reach out to area health professionals as they try to connect to hospice for their patients.

We serve an eight-county area, and as Executive Director of the hospice agency I have several administrative responsibilities. A typical day is working on staff issues and developing programs that will advance the hospice concept in West Virginia.

What advice would you give to someone contemplating the same career path in nursing?

I think hospice nursing is one of the best, if not the best job I have ever had. It offers so much—teaching, networking, reaching out to families, immediate rewards, flexible schedule. If my staff has a Halloween Party for their child at 1 P.M.—they attend that—family is valued. It offers independence and community outreach, a variety that keeps nurses in nursing.

How do you balance career and other aspects of your life?

This is a very hard question—because when you live in a rural area, and work in hospice—I became hospice. It is not a typical job. Because of the extensive outreach—people view you as a missionary almost. I was the first full-time employee at hospice so I really spent a lot of time growing the program. When I started at hospice, it was just me. I did home visits, worked with volunteers, made bereavement calls, did fundraising—my husband became a hospice husband. Now, I realize there is tomorrow—and things will be there. I also found hospice touching all the other aspects of my life—church, community, and so forth.

Do you have any other advice for other nurses who might want to pursue this type of nursing career?

I would say to nurses thinking about a career in hospice to work in a hospital, home health, and then go to hospice. Because once you go to hospice, you will never want to do anything else.

Do you have any other advice for us in preparing this book?

My advice would be just a few comments—one of the pitfalls I feel we have as a nursing profession is that most nurses have not been managed well. I think every nurse should have to take a management course—and this should be part of curriculums of nursing school. In my first job, I thought I had made a grave error by choosing to be a nurse. If nursing was inflexibility, back biting, complaining constantly—I hated nursing. I immediately started working on another degree—an MBA. It was actually the business school professors who showed me it was not nursing I hated—or my job—I just was not managed well. It is through conflict management that we teach each other how to solve problems and work with different personalities.

Infection Control Nurse

1. **Basic description**—Nurse who specializes in identifying, controlling, and preventing outbreaks of infection in health care settings and the community. These nurses establish and implement guidelines directed toward the prevention, detection, and control of infectious processes. Activities include the collection and analysis of infection control data; the planning, implementation, and evaluation of infection prevention and control measures; the education of individuals about infection risk, prevention, and control; the development and revision of infection control policies and procedures; the investigation of suspected outbreaks of infection; and the provision of consultation on infection risk assessment, prevention, and control strategies. Practice areas include long-term care facilities, community or regional hospitals, non-acute inpatient institutions, industry private and public settings, nursing homes, and mental health facilities.

2. **Educational requirements**—RN preparation and BSN required; documented educational programs related to epidemiology, sterilization, sanitation, disinfection, patient care practice, and adult education principles. Certification as an Infection Control Practitioner preferred. Education at MSN or MPH may be required.

3. **Core competencies/skills needed:**
   - Ability to diagnose HIV/AIDS, TB, scabies, nosocomial infections, and other infectious diseases
   - Knowledge of prevention of infectious diseases
   - Knowledge and expertise in microbiology, epidemiology, statistics, sterilization and disinfection, infectious diseases, and antibiotic usage

- Consultative and teaching skills
- Knowledge of the multitude of federal and organizational mandates

4. **Compensation**—Varies with place of employment and geographic location.

5. **Employment outlook**—High

6. **Related Web sites and professional organizations:**
   - Centers for Disease Control and Prevention: www.cdc.gov
   - Association for Professionals in Infection Control and Epidemiology, Inc. (APIC): www.apic.org

Informatics Specialist

1. **Basic description**—Informatics nursing is the integration of nursing and its information management with information processing and communication technology to support the health of people worldwide. Nursing informatics is the specialty that integrates science, computer science, and information science in identifying, collecting, processing, and managing data and information to support nursing practice, administration, research, and the expansion of nursing knowledge. Nursing informatics is currently seen by many executives as a way to improve quality of care and cut costs. Informatics nurses work in a variety of settings such as hospitals, clinics, educational settings, and private consulting firms.

2. **Educational requirements**—BSN degree. Credentialing is available through the American Nurses Credentialing Center.

3. **Core competencies/skills needed:**
   - Ability to conduct major analyses of information
   - Skill in developing data analysis systems and methodologies

- Consultation skills regarding the use of technology
- Marketing skills
- Skill in developing and disseminating reports to staff about cost and other trends in health care
- Ability to use various resources to analyze and interpret variances and make comparisons with national and regional benchmarks
- Ability to manage multiple priorities
- Ability to work independently

4. **Compensation**—Varies with place of employment and geographic location.

5. **Employment outlook**—High

6. **Related Web sites and professional organizations:**
   - American Medical Informatics Association: Nursing Informatics Working Group: www.amia-niwg.org
   - American Nurses Credentialing Center: www.nursingworld.org/ancc
   - American Nursing Informatics Association (ANIA): www.ania.org/

Infusion Therapy Nurse

1. **Basic description**—An infusion nurse has expertise in the field of infusion therapy. The infusion nurse's role is to perform intravenous therapy as well as patient education regarding the task being performed. There are opportunities for infusion therapy nurses to work in hospitals, home care, and various alternative settings such as hospice or long-term care facilities.

2. **Educational requirements**—RN preparation.

3. **Core competencies/skills needed:**
   - Skill in venipuncture

- Knowledge of ways to insure quality care to patients
- Knowledge of nosocomial infection rates and prevention
- Good interpersonal skills

4. **Compensation**—Varies with place of employment and geographic location.
5. **Employment outlook**—Moderate
6. **Related Web site and professional organization:**

- Infusion Nurses Society (INS): www.ins1.org

International Health Nurse

1. **Basic description**—An international health nurse may work on a wide range of global health issues in a number of settings. They may be employed by government agencies [e.g., the United Nations, the World Health Organization, or non-governmental organizations (NGOs)]. They also could be independent consultants. The topics of importance to global nursing include the increasing disparity in access to health care; the growing population of poor (more than one billion people do not have access to basic health and social care, regardless of availability); the rapid environmental changes and degradation of the environment; economic recession and crises in parts of the world that affect the financing of health care; the inability of technology to face epidemics and deadly threats from diseases such as HIV/AIDS, malaria, and tuberculosis; the growing crises and emergencies such as internal conflicts, civil wars, and natural disasters that affect the health delivery systems and access to care.

   International Health Nurses are committed to care for all persons across the life cycle—pregnant women, infants, children, adolescents, adults, and the elderly—and especially vulnerable groups—the poor, refugees and displaced persons, street children, and the homeless.

In setting the future directions for global health policy, nursing and midwifery are key elements. As nurses and midwives already constitute up to 80% of the qualified health workforce in most national health systems, they represent a potentially powerful force for bringing about the necessary changes to meet the needs of health for all in the 21st century. Their contribution to health services covers the whole spectrum of health care, promotion and prevention, as well as health research, planning, implementation, and innovation.

2. **Educational requirements**—RN licensure; graduate preparation in nursing or public health is desirable.
3. **Core competencies/skills needed:**
   - Knowledge of major global health risks such as HIV/AIDS, tuberculosis, smoking, and environmental hazards
   - Knowledge of epidemiology
   - Skills in community mobilization for integrated health development
   - Immunization knowledge and skills
   - Leadership skills
   - Skills in preparing nurses to be ready for emergencies and crisis situations
   - Disaster planning and intervention skills
   - Ability to enhance team building and leadership abilities of nurses as health care providers and planners
   - Public health knowledge
   - Skill in demonstrating cost-effective care through primary health care and the critical role of nurses in the health care team
4. **Compensation**—Varies with place of employment and geographic location.
5. **Employment outlook**—Moderate
6. **Related Web sites and professional organizations:**
   - World Health Organization (WHO): www.who.int/homepage/index.en.shtml
   - International Council of Nurses: www.icn.ch/index.html
   - The Transcultural Nursing Society: www.tcns.org

Inventor

1. **Basic description**—Nurse inventors are those who seek solutions to patient care problems or delivery system problems by creating new devices; often these inventions are patented.
2. **Educational requirements**—RN preparation.
3. **Core competencies/skills needed:**
   - Must possess a desire to fix a problem that has arisen
   - Desire to improve patient and nursing care
   - Creativity
   - Risk-taking skills
   - Tenacity
   - Innovative
   - Belief in your product
4. **Compensation**—Varies with place of employment; may be self-determined.
5. **Employment outlook**—Moderate
6. **Related Web sites and professional organizations:**
   - United States Patent and Trademark Office: www.uspto.gov
   - www.healthcareinventions.com

Lactation Counselor

1. **Basic description**—Lactation consultants and breast-feeding counselors work closely together when a mother is experiencing a breast-feeding problem. They assess the mother and baby, take a history, observe the mother and baby while breast-feeding, problem solve, develop a plan of care, work with and report to the mother's and baby's primary care providers, and arrange for follow-up.

2. **Educational requirements**—The term "lactation consultant" refers to anyone who is working in the field of lactation, either as a volunteer or as a professional. However, certification to become an International Board Certified Lactation Consultant (IBCLC) is considered the gold standard for lactation consultant. This exam is held once a year worldwide. Criteria that must be met for certification are bachelor's, master's, or doctoral degree—or 4 years of post-secondary education; a minimum of 2,500 hours of practice as a breastfeeding consultant; and a minimum of education specific to breast-feeding within the 3 years prior to the exam.

3. **Core competencies/skills needed:**
   - Excellent interpersonal skills
   - Peer counseling skills
   - Excellent knowledge of lactation and women's health

4. **Compensation**—Varies with place of employment and geographic location.

5. **Employment outlook**—Moderate

6. **Related Web sites and professional organizations:**
   - International Lactation Consultant Association (ILCA): www.ilca.org
   - La Leche League International: www.lalecheleague.org

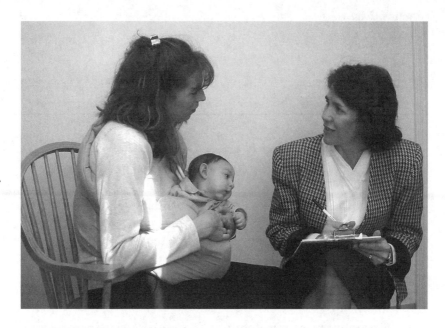

Suzanne Campbell, consulting with mother and baby.

An Interview with
Suzanne Hetzel Campbell,
Lactation Consultant

What is your educational background in nursing (and other areas) and what formal credentials do you hold?

I have the following educational background and certifications: a PhD in Nursing from the University of Rhode Island; a post-master's certificate in Women's Health Advanced Practice Nurse from Boston College; an MS in Nursing from the University of Connecticut; a BS in Nursing from the University of Connecticut, Storrs.

I have the following certifications: IBCLC, International Board Certified Lactation Consultant; Women's Health Care Nurse Practitioner; Licensed as an APRN in the State of Connecticut.

My career has been focused on the area of women's health. I have worked as a staff nurse in obstetrics and gynecology, school nurse, camp nurse, as a breast-feeding aid sales representative, and as a faculty member. I am currently practicing as a Women's Health Nurse Practitioner and work with women experiencing lactation difficulties. This includes making a nursing diagnosis, developing a treatment plan, and follow-up/evaluation. I also have prescriptive privileges. I have various professional memberships and often present at conferences on breast-feeding topics.

How did you first become interested in your current career?

I became interested in nursing my freshman year at the University of Connecticut when I was a biology and pre-med major. I learned about "nurse-midwives" and thought, *that's what I want to do!* I think I was a "researcher" at heart, and so the honors program provided opportunities for that all along the way, culminating in an honor's thesis my senior year, as well as a master's thesis. I worked full-time at the UConn Health Center (UCHC) on a high-risk ob/gyn unit, while working part-time on my master's degree, with a maternal-child focus in the "role of teacher." I did a clinical practicum with a nurse-midwife and student-taught as part of my master's degree program and found that I loved postpartum and working with new mothers at breast-feeding. During my 2 years at UCHC I was surrounded by a very "breast-feeding-supportive" staff. Yet, I think that I did not learn anything about breast-feeding until I had my own child, and it was in my own difficulty those first 6 weeks that I realized how little I knew about everything to do with childbirth, child rearing, and lactation. With La Leche League Leader's support, I trusted my instinct and spent much time "learning in the field." At this point I pursued my doctorate part-time, and focused on breastfeeding as my area of research and clinical expertise. In the years I functioned as a La Leche League Leader, my nursing skills enhanced my ability to help mothers. I found a clinical area that was crying for research, providing me much personal satisfaction in the assistance I was giving others—my niche.

What are the most rewarding aspects of your career?

I enjoy working with new mothers and providing tangible support and seeing the results—being with women "where they are" and helping them discern "who they are." Also, my schedule has the flexibility to meet my own family's needs. I get satisfaction from making the world a better place to live in, just one mother and one baby at a time.

Describe a typical workday in your current position.

I arrive in the office at 9:30 A.M. and switch over from answering service to office phone. Next, I look at the schedule to see patients coming in and look over charts. I meet mother/partner and infant and take into the examining room, where I disappear with them for the next $1\frac{1}{2}$ to 2 hours. I perform a thorough mother/infant history—past, present, physical, etc. I evaluate the breast-feeding relationship, watch a nursing session, and assist with positioning, reading cues, and manual milk expression (by hand or with a pump). Most of the visit is spent in education and counseling; many parenting issues arise as well as breast-feeding, and somehow they are all intermingled. In a typical day, I can see up to four patients, return three to four phone calls, call in prescriptions for antibiotics and antifungals for mother and infant, and do a good amount of confidence boosting. Women who walk into our office are often ready to give up—not just on breast-feeding—on their view of themselves as capable mothers, capable women . . . and we do not convince them all that continued breast-feeding is the right answer. The answer lies within themselves, we just help them understand what is fixable in regard to breast-feeding and help them believe in themselves and their infants.

What advice would you give to someone contemplating the same career path in nursing?

Get as much exposure to your "population" as possible. If you enjoy working with breast-feeding women, DO join the local La Leche League groups to see and hear everything we don't have time to find out in the hospital and the doctors' offices. Recognize there is not a lot of money in this position, but there is the potential for much independence—especially with a combination of APRN/IBCLC. Also recognize the "hours" necessary to gain the clinical expertise for this position and the importance of key mentors (for me Dr. Christina Smillie, MD, FAAP, IBCLC).

How do you balance career and other aspects of your life?

This is a constant challenge! One aspect I appreciate is my exposure to La Leche League very early in my career—a book titled *Sequencing* by Arlene Rossen Cardozo talked about having it all, but not all at once. I learned early that my infant and young child needed me close, so continuing my education, working part-time, and learning as a La Leche League leader in touch with my "postpartum" population through weekly/monthly meetings and telephone counseling—not to mention all the continuing education—kept my hands in my field. Now with older children it remains a challenge, but a supportive spouse and children who have grown in their ability to care for themselves, as well as the help of family and friends close by, makes a difference. Friends who helped me care for my children when they were younger were irreplaceable assets. Finding time even now for friends and family is important. Finding that balance of self-care, which allows exercise, healthful eating, and spiritual tending, is all key to maintaining one's perspective, and one's career.

Do you have any advice for nurses who might want to pursue this type of nursing career?

Lactation consultation is a growing field and becoming an IBCLC has been a dream of mine for the past 10 years. Finding the time to put all the pieces together to achieve it was the trick . . . and achieving my NP first was important. (LCs alone are not reimbursable by third-party payers in CT as NPs are.) I believe (perhaps naïvely) that as research continues to show the multifaceted health benefits of breast-feeding to mother, child, and society, the overburdened U.S. Health Care System will be forced to find more ways to help women be successful at breast-feeding. Skillfully prepared lactation consultants are a key element to successful breast-feeding.

The following is from a press release I recently received with my official test results:

IBLCE International Board of Lactation Consultant Examiners
Press Release: Falls Church October 11, 2002

A record number of 2,294 lactation professionals successfully completed the rigorous requirements to become International Board Certified Lactation

Consultants (IBCLC). The final step in the process was passing a test administered by the IBLCE to demonstrate knowledge required to provide skilled assistance to nursing mothers. The IBCLC Certification is the gold standard of competency in the lactation field. It is the only official, international credential for those offering breastfeeding and lactation care. A combination of basic training, continuing education, practice and successful completion of the examination assures that the designation "IBCLC" identifies a member of the health care team who possesses specialized skills and knowledge. There are now approximately 14,000 IBCLCs worldwide.

IBLCE-certified nurses, physicians, dieticians, educators, midwives, social workers, lay counselors, and therapists work with mothers to excel in the breastfeeding experience. A mother that breastfeeds can save $1,400 per year on formula, is more likely to bond closely with her child, passes on immunities to her child and recovers more quickly from the weight normally gained during pregnancy. Her likelihood of contracting premenopausal breast cancer or osteoporosis over her lifetime is reduced. Studies have shown that babies that are breastfed have fewer visits to health care providers through age 17. The incidence of otitis media, juvenile diabetes, and other illnesses is reduced, not just during the breastfeeding period but also throughout childhood. Assistance by an IBLCE-accredited professional in the critical first hour after birth improves probability of long-term maintenance of breastfeeding.

IBCLCs are ideally skilled to help provide quality breastfeeding care; develop and implement breastfeeding protocols; improve lactation knowledge and skills of other staff and to help their facilities become accredited under the UNICEF "Baby Friendly" Hospital Initiative.

Candidates for the international exam meet stringent eligibility requirements that demonstrate proficiency and understanding of practical skills, clinical judgment, current research knowledge and attainment of a number of continuing education credits. The IBLCE maintains a National/International Registry for all Registered Lactation Consultants. The Registry is a service to the public, employers and supervisors to determine if a provider is a current IBCLC. The Registry can be accessed through the IBLCE website at www.iblce.org and will be updated with the new IBCLCs on December 1st. For more information, contact the IBLCE at 703-560-7330.

Learning/Developmental Disabilities Nurse

1. **Basic description**—The role of a developmental disability nurse is to assist clients with mental and physical disabilities to live as normal and productive a life as possible. This might mean assisting clients with manual and recognition skills to enable them to carry out tasks related to maintaining activities of daily living or developing comprehensive plans with specific goals and objectives. Developmental disabilities nurses work in sheltered workshops, group homes, long-term care facilities, and schools.

2. **Educational requirements**—RN preparation; certification eligibility is available to RNs with a minimum of 4,000 hours (2 years full-time equivalent) of developmental disabilities nursing practice within the past 5 years.

3. **Core competencies/skills needed:**
   - Compassion and understanding of the total person with a disability
   - Patience
   - Excellent communication skills
   - Understanding of chronic long-term disabilities
   - Counseling skills for families
   - Ability to work with interdisciplinary teams
   - Promotes positive life experiences
   - Provides care for health and social needs
   - Understands physical disabilities and psychological/emotional needs
   - Promotes positive images of people with disabilities
   - Applies clinical and behavioral nursing interventions to meet the special health care needs of the individual

- Acts in the capacity of advocate
- Maximizes the client's potential by referring to appropriate resources
- Manages care by coordinating services

4. **Compensation**—Varies with place of employment and geographic location.

5. **Employment outlook**—Moderate

6. **Related Web site and professional organization:**
   - Developmental Disabilities Nurses Association (DDNA): www.ddna.org/

Legal Consultant

1. **Basic description**—Legal nurse consultants are RNs who use specialized health care knowledge and expertise to consult on medical-related cases. Legal consultants provide a variety of services to attorneys, insurance companies, and hospitals in legal matters where health, illness, or injury are issues, such as personal injury, product liability, medical negligence, toxic torts, workers' compensation, risk management, and fraud and abuse. LNCs assist claims managers with the investigation, evaluation, and management of general and professional liability claims by obtaining, organizing, reviewing, and summarizing pertinent records and documents. They assist in the procurement of expert reviews and evaluation of care, and they provide input into the claims resolution strategy based on evaluations. They support managers with implementation of risk-management activities, all with the objective to control or minimize losses to protect the assets of the corporation. Other responsibilities include drafting litigation documents, conducting medical and legal research, · analyzing medical records in depth, and assisting claims manager

with investigation of general and professional liability claims. Employment opportunities are available in law firms, hospitals, insurance companies, government agencies, consulting firms, and self-employment.

2. **Educational requirements**—RN preparation.

3. **Core competencies/skills needed:**
   - Clinical experience required, preferably in a high-risk area
   - Statistical background/data management experience preferred
   - Liability claims/paralegal experience or educational equivalent also preferred
   - Ability to work independently
   - Ability to be a self-starter
   - Comfortable making decisions
   - Excellent reading and writing skills
   - Confidence to talk with experts

4. **Compensation**—Depends on place of employment and geographic location.

5. **Employment outlook**—High

6. **Related Web sites and professional organizations:**
   - American Association of Legal Nurse Consultants: www.aalnc.org
   - The American Association of Nurse Attorneys (TAANA): www.taana.org
   - Medical-Legal Consulting Institute, Inc.: www.legalnurse.com

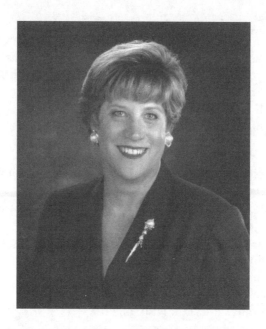

Susan Comstock, Legal Nurse Consultant.

An Interview with Susan Comstock, Legal Nurse Consultant

What is your educational background in nursing (and other areas) and what formal credentials do you hold?

I expect to receive my Doctorate of Nursing (ND) degree in 2003 from Case Western Reserve University. I currently have the following credentials: MS in Nursing; concentration in Nurse-Midwifery; minor in Management from Georgetown University; BS in Nursing from the University of the State of New York, Regents; AD in Nursing from De Anza College; AB in Psychology from Stanford University.

I was involved in maternal/child health as a community activist, birth assistant, and doula before becoming a perinatal nurse. When I became a nurse I joined a Nurse-Midwifery Integration (residency) program and have worked as a Certified Nurse-Midwife since 1987. My experiences range from a solo, private practice, to a teen clinic, to women's health clinics serving vulnerable populations. I have had many years of teaching experience as an assistant professor, lecturer, and clinical instructor and have also worked as a certified childbirth educator and lactation consultant. Since 1997, I have been working as a legal consultant in a medical-legal consulting business I founded, which provides customized services to attorneys, the insurance industry, and government agencies in the areas of medical malpractice, product liability, and general negligence.

How did you first become interested in your current career?

I was appointed to the OB-GYN Quality Improvement Committee at the hospital where I worked and became privy to problems other providers were having in patient care management, as well as systems issues that were a potential medical-legal risk.

What are the most rewarding aspects of your career?

As an independent legal nurse consultant, I get to "call them as I see them." It is very gratifying to be able to keep non-meritorious medical and nursing malpractice lawsuits out of the courts. Additionally, it is rewarding to assist patients and their families who have suffered a severe loss due to egregious malpractice.

Describe a typical workday in your current position.

Fully 20% of my time is spent on business issues, including billing, taxes, marketing, and follow-up activities, including giving legal continuing education lectures at local bar association meetings and chapter activities of the legal nurse consulting group. These are non-billable hours. Another 20% of the time is spent supervising and reviewing the work product of other legal nurse consultant (LNC) subcontractors. Finding expert witnesses of all types for attorneys makes up 10% of time spent. Twenty percent is spent reviewing medical records, and the bulk of the time, 30%, is spent on research and writing analytical reports.

What advice would you give to someone contemplating the same career path in nursing?

Be extremely well organized and able to meet seemingly impossible deadlines. Seek a mentor in the field, and involve yourself in professional legal nurse consultant organizations and conferences. Obtain certification from one of the national groups. Be aware that most attorneys are looking for nurses solely as expert witnesses for particular cases, and that it is difficult to build a practice as a behind-the-scenes, non-testifying consultant.

How do you balance career and other aspects of your life?

My career is my life right now. I am also enrolled in a nursing doctoral program and am tenure-track faculty in the undergraduate and graduate nursing program of the local university, as well as being involved in international health care. My philosophy of life balance is based on life stages. I was fortunate to be able to stay home with my children when they were small. They are now grown and have left the nest, and I am not yet ready to retire.

Do you have any advice for nurses who might want to pursue this type of nursing career?

Apart from your nursing experience and expertise in your field, your success will depend upon your marketing and networking skills, business acumen, and oral and written communication and persuasion abilities. In addition, you must be able to work with attorneys, some of whom can be difficult and challenging. Rather than cutthroat competition with other LNC's, be proactive in establishing cooperative "win-win" relationships. Keep your ethics and integrity intact. Remember that, as a nurse, your first responsibility is to the patient, whether defined as an individual, family, or community.

Long-Term Care Nurse

1. **Basic description**—The long-term care nurse works in a long term care facility with patients with chronic physical and/or mental disorders, who are primarily elderly. Responsible for the day-to-day care of patients, operation of the facility, staff supervision, assessing program quality, program growth and development, and service excellence often are responsibilities of the long-term care nurse. Working in long term care requires working with patients with challenging diagnoses. Practice settings include nursing homes and skilled nursing facilities (SNF).

2. **Educational requirements**—RN preparation.

3. **Core competencies/skills needed:**
   - Prior experience with long-term care
   - Medical and surgical nursing experience
   - Ability to see death as a part of the natural process of life
   - Ability to build long-term relationships with patients and their families
   - Ability to build teams and mentor others
   - Leadership and organizational ability
   - Ability to solve staffing difficulties when they arise

4. **Compensation**—Varies with place of employment and geographic location.

5. **Employment outlook**—High

6. **Related Web site and professional organization:**
   - American Long Term and Sub Acute Nurses Association: www.alsna.com

Media Consultant

1. **Basic description**—Nurses who are media consultants provide behind the scenes and up-front consultation for media in order to present accurate and realistic portrayals of health care, patient care, and the professional practice of nursing.

2. **Educational requirements**—RN preparation but often RNs with advanced degrees and certifications in their specialty fields are preferred.

3. **Core competencies/skills needed:**
    - Knowledge of television, movie, and stage environments
    - Ability to work with a wide variety of individuals from producers to actors
    - Ability to work with deadlines
    - Ability to work in a fast-paced, rapidly changing environment

4. **Compensation**—Varies with assignment.

5. **Employment outlook**—Moderate

6. **Related Web sites and professional organizations:**
    - Registered Nurse Experts, Inc.: www.rnexperts.com
    - Sigma Theta Tau International—media guide

Medical Records Auditor

1. **Basic description**—A medical records auditor audits, examines, verifies, adjusts, and corrects medical records and bills to ensure accuracy and consistency. They report discrepancies to personnel and ensure corrective action is taken in a timely manner. They audit physician billing practices against documentation in the medical record to ensure compliance with all federal, state, and third-party billing requirements, rules, and regulations. Medical records auditors go through medical records to make sure everything is in compliance and all the codes match up for billing purposes.

2. **Educational requirements**—RN preparation. Many facilities also prefer that the applicant has some college level business courses or health care experience.

3. **Core competencies/skills needed:**
    *   Strong analytical skills and some basic training skills to teach people how to correct problems
    *   A basic knowledge of diagnostic related groups (DRGs) and coding
    *   A broad knowledge of disease process, findings, course of treatment, quality assurance, and risk management are essential

4. **Compensation**—Varies with place of employment and geographic location.

5. **Employment outlook**—High

6. **Related Web sites and professional organizations:**
    *   National Committee for Quality Assurance: www.ncqa.org/
    *   Agency for Healthcare Research and Quality: www.ahrq.gov/
    *   National Association for Healthcare Quality: www.nahq.org/

Medical–Surgical Nurse

1. **Basic description**—Medical–surgical nurses are Registered nurses (RNs) who specialize in the care of patients admitted with nonsurgical (medical) and surgical conditions. These nurses work to promote health, prevent disease, and help patients cope with illness. They are advocates and health educators for patients, families, and communities. The medical-surgical nurse has an incredibly complex job. The entry-level medical-surgical nurse makes nursing judgments based on scientific knowledge and relies on procedures and standardized care plans. Nursing care is directed toward alleviating physical and psychosocial health problems. Advancing to an intermediate level, the medical-surgical nurse with experience becomes more skilled in developing individual and innovative care plans to meet client needs. With a broader base of experience, a more advanced clinician cares for clients with complex and unpredictable problems. The most common place of employment is the hospital.

2. **Educational requirements**—RN preparation; often requires MSN preparation. Certification is available through ANCC.

3. **Core competencies/skills needed:**
   - Excellent observation and assessment skills
   - Skill in recording symptoms, reactions, and progress
   - Skill in administering medical treatments and examinations
   - Knowledge of convalescence and rehabilitation requirements for patients
   - Skill in developing, planning, implementing, evaluating, documenting, and managing nursing care
   - Patient and family education
   - Ability to help individuals and groups take steps to improve or maintain their health

4. **Compensation**—Varies with place of employment and geo-graphic location.

5. **Employment outlook**—High

6. **Related Web sites and professional organizations:**
   - Academy of Medical-Surgical Nurses: http://amsn.inurse.com/
   - American Nurses Credentialing Exam: www.nursingworld.org/ancc/

Neonatal Nurse Practitioner

1. **Basic description**—Neonatal nurse practitioners are advanced practice nurses who specialize in providing care to acutely ill babies in the neonatal intensive care unit (NICU). These nurses have advanced skills in physical and psychosocial assessment of the newborn and handle transport of acutely ill babies. The environments in which neonatal nurse practitioners work are very intense and dramatic often with non-stop action.

2. **Educational requirements**—RN preparation and MSN with advanced practice certification as a neonatal nurse practitioner. Programs are generally 2 years in length. These programs are affiliated with major medical centers that are equipped to care for premature babies. Previous experience in the NICU is usually a requirement for admission to a neonatal nurse practitioner pro-gram.

3. **Core competencies/skills needed:**
   - Technical competency involving use of complex and compu-terized equipment
   - Skill in regulating ventilators
   - Hemodynamic monitoring skills

- Experiences and expertise in assessing and managing acutely ill babies
- Skill in obtaining blood samples from central IV lines
- Interpersonal competency dealing with patients and their families in life-threatening situations
- Ability to work with interdisciplinary teams
- Ability to support parents' decisions even when you do not agree
- Comfort working with very small babies
- Ability to support a parents decision even when you do not agree

4. **Compensation**—Salaries vary according to place of employment and geographic location. The average is $62,000 to $80,000 but can be much higher depending on level of responsibility.

5. **Employment outlook**—High

6. **Related Web sites and professional organizations:**
   - American Association of Nurse Practitioners: www.aanp.org
   - Nurse Practitioner Support Services: www.nurse.net
   - Pediatric Critical Care Medicine: www.pedsccm.wust1.edu
   - Association of Women's Health, Obstetric and Neonatal Nurses (AWHONN): www.awhonn.org/
   - National Association of Neonatal Nurses (NANN): www.nann.org/
   - American Nurse Association Credentialing Center: www.ana.org

---

Nephrology Nurse

1. **Basic description**—A nephrology nurse works with patients who have acute or chronic renal failure. The nurse works with patients in all stages of renal disease, as well as administers

treatment such as peritoneal dialysis and hemodialysis in a variety of settings. Examples of places of employment include hospitals, outpatient clinics, dialysis settings, and patients' homes.

2. **Educational requirements**—RN preparation. Although not a requirement for employment, a certification in dialysis nursing is helpful. On-the-job training is a large part of becoming adept at dialysis nursing. It takes approximately 6 weeks to train a nurse with experience and about 6 months before nurses are truly comfortable and able to troubleshoot problems effectively.

3. **Core competencies/skills needed:**
   - Ability to assess even very subtle changes in the condition of a dialysis/nephrology patient
   - Ability to understand and operate equipment used for hemo-dialysis
   - Excellent interpersonal and communication skills, especially when working with patients and their families as they deal with chronic renal disease and its impact
   - Ability to teach patient about renal disease, treatment, and lifestyle changes
   - Ability to deal with grief and loss that can be associated with renal disease
   - Collaboration and teamwork

4. **Compensation**—Vary according to place of employment and geographic location, but generally do not differ from wages for staff nurses on other units.

5. **Employment outlook**—High

6. **Related Web site and professional organization:**
   - American Nephrology Nurses' Association (ANNA): www.annanurse.org

Neuroscience Nurse

1. **Basic description**—Neuroscience nurses take care of individuals who have experienced changes in function or alterations in consciousness and cognition communication, mobility, rest and sleep, sensations, and sexuality. A nurse working in the neuroscience field should enjoy technology and working with people, and have both physical and psychological stamina.

2. **Educational requirements**—RN preparation.

3. **Core competencies/skills needed:**
   - Skills in patient and family education, especially regarding the neurological condition
   - Skill in using the nursing process to plan and implement care
   - Knowledge of neuroscience nursing, including anatomy and physiology, illness manifestations, and medical treatments
   - Ability to manage families and individuals who are grieving loss
   - Technological skills

4. **Compensation**—Varies with place of employment and geographic location.

5. **Employment outlook**—High

6. **Related Web sites and professional organizations:**
   - American Association of Neuroscience Nurses: www.aann.org
   - American Association of Spinal Cord Injury Nurses: www.aascin.org

Nurse Anesthetist

1. **Basic description**—Nurse anesthetists are responsible for inducing anesthesia, maintaining it at the required levels, and supporting life functions while anesthesia is being administered. Nurse anesthetists administer all types of anesthesia and may perform general, local, and regional anesthesia procedures to pediatric, adult, and geriatric patients, using invasive monitoring techniques when necessary. These nurses practice as part of a highly skilled interdisciplinary team. A variety of practice settings exist including

   - Emergency rooms
   - Operating rooms
   - Physicians' offices
   - Plastic surgery practices
   - Dental practices
   - Orthopedic practices

2. **Educational requirements**—RN preparation with CRNA certification; MSN preferred. To enter a nurse anesthetist program, one must possess an active RN license and a baccalaureate degree (may or may not be in nursing). The person must also fulfill certain prerequisites before applying which vary according to institution. The applicant must also possess a minimum of 1 year of critical care experience as an RN.

3. **Core competencies/skills needed:**

   - Assessment skills and a constant awareness of what is going on at all times
   - Skill in history taking and physical assessment
   - Patient education skills

- Ability to recognize and take appropriate corrective action (including consulting with anesthesiologist) for abnormal patient responses
- Excellent observation skills
- Ability to provide resuscitative care until the patient has regained control of vital functions
- Skill in administering spinal, epidural, auxiliary, and field blocks

4. **Compensation**—Average starting salaries are in the high $70,000s, but there is a considerable range depending on the place of employment and willingness to be on call for emergency cases.

5. **Employment outlook**—High

6. **Related Web sites and professional organizations:**

- American Association of Nurse Anesthetists (AANA): www.aana.com
- Council on Certification of Nurse Anesthetists

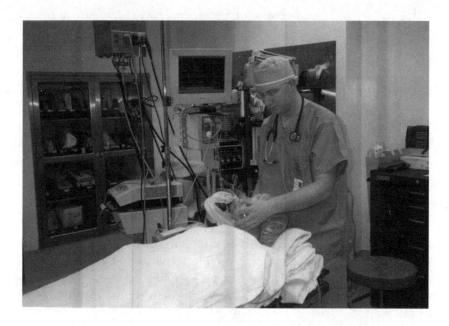

Christopher Reinhart, at work as a Nurse Anesthetist.

An Interview with Christopher Reinhart, Nurse Anesthetist

What is your educational background in nursing (and other areas) and what formal credentials do you hold?

I have the following credentials: MSN with a major in nurse anesthesia; BSN degree; and an RN diploma program.

My certifications include ACLS (Advanced Cardiac Life Support); BCLS (Basic Cardiac Life Support); PALS (Pediatric Advanced Life Support); NRP (Neonatal Resuscitation Program); and EMT-P (Paramedic).

How did you first become interested in your current career?

A career in nurse anesthesia has interested me since I was in my 2-year RN program. After working in critical care nursing areas for 5 years, I wanted additional responsibility in a different type of critical care environment. After exploring several options, I chose nurse anesthesia. Before choosing the nurse anesthetist program, I shadowed nurse anesthetists and interviewed a few of them.

What are the most rewarding aspects of your career?

Having the ability to calm nervous patients and tend to their needs while they are under anesthesia; having the knowledge and ability to relieve a laboring mother's pain shortly after meeting her; and obtaining respect from my colleagues. I love doing the job I do and the results of my work are frequently instantaneous.

Describe a typical workday in your current position.

I currently work two 8-hour shifts 7 to 3:30 in general surgery and one 24-hour shift in obstetric anesthesia every week. In general surgery, I arrive at 7:00 A.M., pick up my assignment, draw up medications, and set up my anesthesia machine and equipment. I then interview my first patient, perform a brief history and physical and discuss my anesthesia plan with the patient. I provide anesthesia to the patient from start to finish and then transfer the patient to the post anesthesia care unit. This process repeats itself two to six times per day depending on the length of cases.

In obstetrics, I work a 24-hour shift. I get called for the placement of epidurals in mothers who request them and I perform spinals on C-section cases. I also cover the entire hospital for emergency intubations.

What advice would you give to someone contemplating the same career path in nursing?

Strive to get the highest GPA possible in your undergraduate preparations. Work in an adult ICU at a large hospital for 1-year minimum. (Several years or more can increase your chance of being accepted.) Visit the AANA website at www.aana.com for more information. Shadow a CRNA for several days. Interview CRNAs and student nurse anesthetists. Call a school of nurse anesthesia for their information brochure. Call 1-847-692-7050 for a flier on the CRNA profession from the AANA (American Association of Nurse Anesthetists).

How do you balance career and other aspects of your life?

Flexible scheduling allows for many days off and ample vacation time depending on where you work. CRNAs can often choose between a combination of 8, 10, 12, or 24-hour shifts. CRNAs can commonly start a new job with 4 to 5 weeks of vacation per year plus 1 week off for continuing education classes. For CRNAs who do not want to work full-time, many options are available to work part-time or as needed.

Do you have any advice for nurses who might want to pursue this type of nursing career?

Acceptance into a CRNA program is very competitive and the number of applicants continues to rise. To increase your chances of getting accepted, strive to get the best grades possible in your undergraduate preparations, and continue working an adult ICU setting. In addition, make sure before enrolling that becoming a CRNA is right for you. Talk with a few CRNAs and shadow CRNAs at least twice in different areas to see what they do. The job of a CRNA can be routine at times, however, a patient's condition can deteriorate at a moment's notice requiring critical thinking and rapid interventions from the CRNA. Depending on where a CRNA works, you may work independently, or as part of an anesthesia team.

Nurse Midwife

1. **Basic description** — Certified nurse midwives are advance practice nurses who specialize in providing care to healthy women during pregnancy, childbirth, and after birth. Nurse midwives may specialize in obstetrics or women's wellness. Midwives provide accessible, safe birth care especially in rural and inner city areas where obstetricians are often less available. They teach patients and their families about the birthing process and often provide the mother in labor more birthing information and individualized attention. They provide care in a variety of settings including hospitals, birthing centers, clinics, homes, and offices.

2. **Educational requirements** — RN preparation plus a baccalaureate degree (not necessarily in nursing) are required to become a nurse midwife. There are prerequisites that must be met, but vary from one organization to another. The typical program averages 12 months and a master's degree is the usual degree earned. The certification examination for nurse midwives is offered through the American College of Nurse-Midwives Certification Council.

3. **Core competencies/skills needed:**
   - Strong assessment skills specifically related to this specialty
   - Good communication ability
   - Excellent leadership and organizational skills
   - Understanding of relevant technology
   - Ability to collaborate with other members of the health care team
   - Compassion and caring attitude
   - Ability to deal with a variety of people

4. **Compensation** — The salary range is approximately $40,000 to $110,000 per year.

5. **Employment outlooks**—High
6. **Related Web sites and professional organizations:**
   - American College of Nurse-Midwives: www.acnm.org or www.midwife.org
   - The ACNM Certification Council (ACC): www.accmidwife.org
   - Association of Women's Health, Obstetrics and Neonatal Nurses (AWHONN): www.awhonn.org

---

Nurse Psychotherapist

1. **Basic description**—Nurse psychotherapists work in a therapeutic relationship with their patients on either a one-to-one basis or in small therapy groups. Therapists form therapeutic alliances with their patients in order to help them to decrease their symptoms and to return to pre-illness level of function. Nurse psychotherapists work in a variety of settings including hospitals, clinics, and independent practice.

2. **Educational requirements**—RN preparation plus a master's degree and preparation as an advanced practice nurse. National certification by the ANCC in specialty.

3. **Core competencies/skills needed:**
   - Advanced clinical skills in the area of psychiatric/mental health nursing
   - Ability to practice independently in areas such as medication management and psychotherapy
   - Ability to integrate research and theory into the practice of psychotherapy
   - Ability to provide individual psychotherapy and psychiatric assessment

- Ability to integrate nursing science, computer science, and informatics in the provision of care
- Works collaboratively with other specialty groups

4. **Compensation**—Varies with place of employment and geographic location in the hospital setting; independent practice consultation $120 to $150 per hour.

5. **Employment outlook**—High

6. **Related Web sites and professional organizations:**
   - American Psychiatric Nurses Association: www.acapn.org
   - Society for Education and Research in Psychiatric Mental Health Nursing: www.serpn2aol.com

---

Nutrition Support Nurse

1. **Basic description**—Nutrition support nurses play a major role in the maintenance of patients' nutritional health. While most patients are able to eat or may just require some encouragement and assistance, some patients are unable to meet their nutritional needs via the oral route. The provision of nutrition support, which includes enteral feeding (via the gastrointestinal tract) and total parenteral nutrition (via the venous circulation), allows maintenance or repletion of the nutritional status for this group of patients. Nutrition support is provided by a multidisciplinary team comprising nurse clinicians, dieticians, gastroenterologists, surgeons, and pharmacists. The nurse clinician and team coordinate, provide, and advise patients on nutrition support. The team ensures that patients' nutritional needs are met by the safest, most economical and efficacious nutritional modality. Often the work includes assistance for children who require special nutritional intervention, including those with feeding disorders, growth failure, dietary intolerance, short bowel syndrome and

congenital bowel disorders, and malabsorption. Nutrition support services can be provided to administer long-term intravenous nutrition or specialized tube feedings in selected cases.

2. **Educational requirements**—RN preparation.

3. **Core competencies/skills needed:**
   - Skill in developing guidelines and protocols on patient nutrition support
   - Ability to manage the various acute and chronic nutritional access devices, both enteral as well as parenteral
   - Skill in developing, implementing, and evaluating appropriate programs for staff training and patient teaching
   - Interdisciplinary team skills
   - Ability to work in a range of health care settings

4. **Compensation**—Varies with place of employment and geographic location.

5. **Employment outlook**—High

6. **Related Web site and professional organization:**
   - American Society for Parenteral and Enteral Nutrition: www.nutritioncare.org/

Occupational/Industrial Nurse

1. **Basic description**—Occupational health nurses work in a variety of settings to keep workers healthy and to prevent work-related injuries. These nurses provide direct care services to employees on the job, host health promotion activities, and provide workers' compensation case management. This nurse is also often responsible for treatment of hazards in specific work environments. Practice settings include businesses, industries, government facilities, and shopping malls.

2. **Educational requirements**—RN preparation; BSN is often preferred and graduate education may be required. Usually 2 years
   of medical/surgical experience is required. To qualify for accreditation exam, $2^1/2$ years of experience or 4,000 hours of patient
   contact are needed.

3. **Core competencies/skills needed:**
   - Knowledge of Occupational Safety & Health Administration
     (OSHA) regulations and workers' compensation laws
   - Ability to maintain, protect, and preserve the health of em-
     ployees in their work environment
   - Ability to analyze and prioritize employee risk factors to
     achieve highest level of health among employees
   - Ability to coordinate care
   - Assist in meeting OSHA standards
   - Ability to provide health education
   - Ability to manage crisis/emergencies
   - Autonomy
   - Innovative thinker
   - Good communication skills
   - Excellent health assessment skills
   - Effective manager

4. **Compensation**—Salary is negotiable depending on state, degree
   held, and company.

5. **Employment outlook**—High

6. **Related Web site and professional organization:**
   - American Association of Occupational Health Nurses, Inc.:
     www.aaohn.org

Office Nurse

1. **Basic description**—Office nurses perform routine administrative and clinical tasks to keep the offices and clinics of family practice physicians, internal medicine, oncologists, cardiologists, surgeons, advanced practice nurses, and others running smoothly. The goal of the office nurse is to provide personalized and efficient service to the patients they serve. They often play an important role in uncovering problems or concerns of the patient and alert the physician to them. They perform telephone triage and provide patient education about many routine topics. They care for the patients in offices, clinics, surgical centers, and emergency medical centers. Depending on the type of facility, the office nurse serves patients with a variety of needs—diagnostic, medication, monitoring, wound treatment, maintenance, preventive medicine, surgery, and education. One of the most important responsibilities of an office nurse is telephone triage, integrating appropriate attention to biologic and psychosocial issues with high-quality medical care. Another vital role for office nurses is that of patient advocate. Duties vary from office to office, depending on location, size, and specialty. Administrative duties often include answering telephones, greeting patients, updating and filing patient medical records, filling out insurance forms, handling correspondence, scheduling appointments, arranging for hospital admission and laboratory services, and handling billing and bookkeeping.

2. **Educational requirements**—RN preparation; experience is often a major requirement, but there are classes available to enhance telephone triage skills.

3. **Core competencies/skills needed:**
   - Good communication skills
   - Knowledge of disease processes and normal development

- Office management skills
- History taking and physical assessment skills
- Patient and family education
- Knowledge of medications
- Skill in routine nursing activities such as dressing changes, vital signs, and assessment

4. **Compensation**—Varies according to place of employment and geographic location.

5. **Employment outlook**—High

6. **Related Web site and professional organization:**

- The American Association of Office Nurses (AAON): www.aaon.org/

Ombudsman

1. **Basic description**—An ombudsman is someone who investigates reported complaints, reports findings, and helps achieve equitable settlements. They handle complaints and concerns regarding the quality of life and the quality of care of vulnerable adults receiving long-term care services. Activities they perform include information and referral, problem solving, conflict resolution, mediation, and education. Because of the nature and diversity of the complaints and concerns, there is a need to work with many state and local organizations. The sources of the complaints are varied from the client themselves, to their families, to provider staff, to doctors, to reps from state agencies, to hospital discharge planners. The complaints range from straightforward to multifaceted. For example, some need specialized equipment, some have restraint concerns. Complaints may also include inadequate staffing, financial exploitation, alleged staff abuse, family conflicts, cold food, lost laundry, poor infection

control, and decubitus ulcers. An ombudsman works with the Department of Health, the regulatory agency for all health care facilities in the long-term care continuum. They are often closely involved with the Departments of Elderly Affairs, Human Services, and Mental Health, Retardation, and hospitals, as they are providers and payers of care to the targeted population. They also work closely with the state's Attorney General's office, attorneys, and the probate court system. As part of an organization, there is involvement in many committees, task forces, and councils, leading to legislative activities.

2. **Educational requirements**—RN preparation: nursing background and experience is of benefit because of many concerns regarding clinical issues. It is also beneficial to have nursing input due to the high acuity levels of people receiving long-term care services along with the dealings with the hospitals, the medical community, and the nursing industry at all levels. Families and clients also feel added reassurance that a nurse is involved.

3. **Core competencies/skills needed:**
    - Excellent listening and interpersonal skills
    - Skill in documentation
    - Flexibility
    - Ability to work with individuals from a variety of backgrounds
    - Management skills required for dealing with a large number of agencies and representatives

4. **Compensation**—Varies according to place of employment and geographic location.

5. **Employment outlook**—Moderate

6. **Related Web sites and professional organizations:**
    - The Ombudsman Association: www.ombuds-toa.org/
    - United States Ombudsman Association: www.usombudsman.org

Oncology Nurse

1. **Basic description**—An oncology nurse cares for patients with cancer in various stages of the disease. Most patients experience problems from both the disease and the treatment. Oncology nurses administer chemotherapy, manage symptoms and the effects of treatment, and care for the needs of their patients with empathy. They must also deal with the psychological ramifications that the diagnosis of cancer brings as well as issues related to death and dying. Oncology nurses may be employed in a variety of settings. They most often work on special oncology units within hospitals, but may work in outpatient areas, home care, and hospice care.

2. **Educational requirements**—RN preparation; a BSN or higher degree in nursing may be required. Some agencies may require certification as an oncology nurse.

3. **Core competencies/skills needed:**
    *   Ability to cope with human suffering, emergencies, and other stresses
    *   Maturity
    *   Excellent interpersonal and communication skills
    *   Strong teaching ability
    *   Able to adapt to new treatment regimens
    *   Knowledge of drugs used in chemotherapy is essential
    *   Strong knowledge background in disease processes and symptom management in particular forms of cancer

4. **Compensation**—Varies according to place of employment and geographic location.

5. **Employment outlook**—High

6. **Related Web sites and professional organizations:**
   - Oncology Nursing Society (ONS): www.ons.org
   - Oncology Nursing Certification Corporation: www.oncc.org
   - Association of Pediatric Oncology Nurses: www.apon.org/

Ophthalmic Nurse

1. **Basic description**—An ophthalmic nurse cares for patients with disorders and disease relating to the eyes. Ophthalmic nursing is full of opportunities for dedicated and highly skilled nurses who want to work with patients with ophthalmic diseases. Although it is a specialized field, it is also a career full of opportunities for nurses who want to use their general nursing knowledge and skills. Work settings include ophthalmologists' offices, hospitals, day surgery centers, research laboratories, and eye banks.
2. **Educational requirements**—RN preparation. The National Certifying Board for Ophthalmic Registered Nurses is an independently incorporated organization supported by the American Society of Ophthalmic Registered Nurses for the purpose of developing and implementing the certifying process for ophthalmic registered nurses. Candidates who meet the following criteria are eligible to take the certification examination for ophthalmic registered nurses: Currently licensed as a registered nurse in the United States or the equivalent hours (4,000) experience in ophthalmic registered nursing practice; completion and filing of an application for certification examination for ophthalmic registered nurses.
3. **Core competencies/skills needed:**
   - Ability to provide psychosocial support for patients and families
   - Excellent communication skills

- Understanding of diseases of the eye and treatment protocols
- Ability to work in the operating room to assist with operative procedures

4. **Compensation**—Varies according to place of employment and geographic location.

5. **Employment outlook**—Moderate

6. **Related Web site and professional organization:**

- American Society of Ophthalmic Registered Nurses (ASORN): www.webeye.ophth.uiowa.edu/asorn/

Organ Donation Counselor

1. **Basic description**—An organ donation specialist/counselor is a nurse who works with families who have loved ones with irrevocable injuries on life support, and discusses the possibility of organ donation. There is a critical shortage of tissue and organ donation for transplants and nurses can play a vital role in eliminating this shortage. Organ donation nurses are highly specialized and there are many related responsibilities. The education of nurses as designated requesters may have a considerable impact on the number of donors, because nurses are close to prospective donors and their families. Nurses provide a vital connection in the organ donation process.

2. **Educational requirements**—RN preparation. There are many programs that educate nurses to become donation requestors. The American Board of Transplant Coordinators (ABTC) offers two certifications to transplant coordinators after working in the field for a minimum of 1 year. Certification is available as either a CPTC (certified procurement transplant coordinator) or a CCTC (certified clinical transplant coordinator).

3. **Core competencies/skills needed:**

- Maturity
- Familiarity with types of donation and donation criteria
- Know the agency policy
- Know the types of transplantations
- Familiarity with different religious positions regarding tissue and organ donation
- Ability to deal with issues related to death and dying

4. **Compensation**—Varies according to place of employment and geographic location.

5. **Employment outlook**—Moderate

6. **Related Web sites and professional organizations:**
   - International Transplant Nurses Society (ITNS): www.itns.org/
   - North American Transplant Coordinators' Organization: www.natco1.org/

OR Nurse/Perioperative Nurse

1. **Basic description**—A perioperative nurse or operating room (OR) nurse is a member of a surgical team that provides care for a patient before, during, and immediately after the patient has experienced a surgical intervention.

2. **Educational requirements**—RN preparation. Certification is available through the Association of Operating Room Nurses (AORN).

3. **Core competencies/skills needed:**
   - Knowledge and skills needed to assist in preparing and operating the technological tools involved in new surgical techniques now available (e.g., lighter fiberoptic scopes/lenses and video monitors)

- Skill in providing comfort measures to the patient
- Skill in assisting the anesthetic caregivers
- Respect for cultural diversity, patients rights, privacy, and confidentiality
- Team skills for interactions with surgeons, surgical technologists, other nurses, anesthesiologists, nurse anesthetists, pathologists, radiologists, perfusionists, support assistant staff, and many other members of the health care team
- Skill in facilitating patient advocacy
- Excellent basic nursing skills in observation and assessment

4. **Compensation**—Varies according to place of employment and geographic location.

5. **Employment outlook**—High

6. **Related Web site and professional organization:**
   - The Association of Perioperative Registered Nurses: www.aorn.org

Orthopedic Nurse

1. **Basic description**—Orthopedic nurses care for patients of all ages with actual and potential muscular skeletal injuries and conditions. An orthopedic nurse may provide assessments and educate patients about braces, prosthetics, and other orthopedic equipment. The nurse must be interested in the care of patients before and after surgery involving the muscular skeletal system such as total hip replacement, arthroscopy, total knee replacement, or spinal surgery. Orthopedic nursing is full of opportunities for dedicated and highly skilled nurses who want to work with patients with orthopedic conditions. Work settings include sports medicine clinics, sports franchises, hospitals, clinics, and day surgery centers.

2. **Educational requirements**—RN preparation. The Orthopaedic Nurses Certification Board provides a credentialing mechanism that validates proficiency in orthopedic nursing practice. Candidates who meet the following criteria are eligible to take the examination: Currently licensed as a registered nurse, 2 years of professional nursing practice, and minimum of 1,000 hours of work experience in orthopedic nursing within the last 3 years.

3. **Core competencies/skills needed:**
   - Excellent communication skills
   - Understanding of the laws of physics
   - Interest in sports and physical activity

4. **Compensation**—Varies according to place of employment and geographic location.

5. **Employment outlook**—Moderate

6. **Related Web site and professional organization:**
   - National Association of Orthopedic Nurses (NAON): www.orthonurse.org

---

Otolaryngology Nurse

1. **Basic description**—The otolaryngology nurse cares for patients with diverse medical and surgical problems relating to disorders of the ear, nose, throat, and other structures of the head and neck. Patients with disorders related to the head and neck frequently present with complex problems because of the visible nature of the condition. The working environment in caring for patients with conditions of the head and neck is very intense. The nurse must continually be involved in assessment, planning, implementation, and evaluation of care. Some of the conditions of these patients are cleft palate, ear and sinus disorders, plastic and reconstructive surgery, and head and neck cancer. Employers

are hospital operating rooms, ambulatory surgery centers, office practices, clinics, schools, and hospice and home care agencies.

2. **Educational requirements**—RN preparation. Certification by the National Certifying Board of Otorhinolaryngology and Head-Neck Nurses (NCBOHN).

3. **Core competencies/skills needed:**
   - Strong medical-surgical nursing background
   - Sound knowledge of anatomy and physiology
   - Sound nutrition and fluid and electrolyte balance background
   - Knowledge of pain management
   - Understanding and empathy of body image alteration
   - Interpersonal competency
   - Ability to work with interdisciplinary teams
   - Knowledge of growth and development across the life span since patients are of all age groups
   - Ability to teach
   - Excellent communication skills including sign language
   - Sensitivity to patient self-image

4. **Compensation**—Varies according to place of employment and geographic location.

5. **Employment outlook**—Moderate

6. **Related Web site and professional organization:**
   - Society of Otorhinolaryngology and Head–Neck Nurses, Inc.: www.sohnnurse.com/

Pain Management Nurse

1. **Basic description**—The pain management nurse collaborates with an interdisciplinary team in the management of patients with acute and chronic pain. Pain management is a Joint Com-

mission on Accreditation standard and is a critical need of many patients. Opportunities exist to work in acute care settings, outpatient clinics, rehabilitation centers, and home care.

2. **Educational requirements**—RN preparation.

3. **Core competencies/skills needed:**
   - Empathy and understanding
   - Understanding of the physiological and psychological aspects of pain
   - Excellent communication skills
   - Ability to work with interdisciplinary teams
   - Interest in the complex issues regarding pain and the control of pain

4. **Compensation**—Varies according to place of employment and geographic location.

5. **Employment outlook**—High

6. **Related Web sites and professional organizations:**
   - Pain Management and Nursing Role/Core Competency: A Guide for Nurses: www.dhmh.state.md.us/mbn/practice/pain_management.pdf
   - American Society of Pain Management Nurses (ASPMN): www.aspmn.org

Parish Nurse

1. **Basic description**—A registered nurse who facilitates the holistic health of a congregation by focusing on spiritual, emotional, and physical dimensions of a person. Parish nurses act as liaison and facilitator between church, community, and hospital and work with clergy in meeting the physical and spiritual needs of members of a particular congregation. Activities of parish nurses

include community screenings (e.g., taking blood pressures, patient teaching, making home visits, and counseling and patient advocacy).

2. **Educational requirements**—RN preparation.

3. **Core competencies/skills needed:**
   - Interest in helping members of a congregation maintain optimum levels of health and independent living
   - Excellent communication skills
   - Caring and compassionate
   - Strong religious affiliation
   - Patient and family education
   - Excellent assessment skills
   - Advocacy skills

4. **Compensation**—Generally, parish nurses serve in a volunteer capacity in hospitals and/or religious organizations and congregations and do not receive monetary compensation.

5. **Employment outlook**—Moderate

6. **Related Web sites and professional organizations:**
   - Health Ministries USA:
     www.pcusa.org/health/usa/parishnursing/parishnursing.htm
   - International Parish Nurse Resource Center:
     http://ipnrc.parishnurses.org/index.phtml
   - North Central Region Health Ministries Network: About Parish Nurses and Health Ministries; Frequently Asked Questions: www.healthministries.net/FAQs.htm

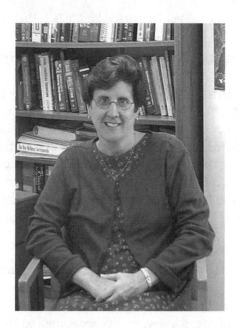

Cindy Drenning, Parish Nurse.

An Interview
with Cindy J. Drenning,
Parish Nurse

What is your educational background in nursing (and other areas) and what formal credentials do you hold?

My educational background is as follows: MSN, Family Nurse Practitioner from West Virginia University; BSN, Nursing from Pennsylvania State University.

I have worked in many aspects of nursing from medical-surgical to community and home health. I also worked as a health consultant and a school nurse before becoming a parish nurse. Currently I am involved in community activities as well as serving as an academic advisor and faculty member.

How did you first become interested in your current career?

I learned about parish nursing from the pastor of the church where I was a member in 1990. This is the same church I am currently serving. He sparked my interest, and I began to read and learn all I could about the role. It rekindled a flame in me that had all but died. I learned to practice whole-person health care and found this difficult in our highly technical health care delivery system. In 1999 when I received my master's degree, I added the advanced practice dimension to my practice. I do not provide primary care to individuals, but work collaboratively with their primary care providers to better address health care concerns.

What are the most rewarding aspects of your career?

It is a privilege to be allowed to enter the lives of individuals and families at times of joy, sorrow, and crisis related to their health state. It is very rewarding when they begin to see the mind–body–spirit link related to their particular health issue. I have learned much from the elderly and oldest–old of the congregation related to healthy spiritual aging. I have also learned much about grief and bereavement from working with individuals going through this process.

Describe a typical workday in your current position.

I will give some examples of things I encounter in the parish nurse role, obviously not all of these occur in one day. I answer many phone calls related to health questions needing referral to community re-sources, and questions from the community resources needing assis-tance from the church. I visit in the home, hospital, nursing home, and my office seeing individuals with physical, emotional, and spiritual health needs. Physical needs most often relate to diabetes, hypertension, or cancer. I am not the primary care provider, but work with the individual to look at the problem holistically and explore what other factors are contributing to the condition. Many physical health issues are in better control when we look at the emotional and spiritual components of health. I provide therapeutic listening to individuals with such mental health issues as depression and anxiety, assisting them in looking at better coping mechanisms and supporting their primary mental health care. Issues related to spiritual distress are addressed and have a profound impact on the well being of the individual.

Health education is a large part of my role and I plan and facilitate or provide health education programs relating to mind–body–spirit health. I write articles for our local newsletter and the state newsletter for our denomination again relating to whole-person health. I coordinate support groups as needed.

What advice would you give to someone contemplating the same career path in nursing?

Examine yourself first and know your own physical, emotional, and spiritual health needs. Know, understand, and respect the care of the whole person—mind, body, and spirit. Know your community, and establish the role with the needs of the faith community and larger community in mind.

How do you balance career and other aspects of your life?

I try to practice holistic self-care, recognizing and providing attention to my own physical, emotional, and spiritual needs. I try also to stay truly in the moment with clients, so that I may leave at the end of the day knowing I gave my very best in whatever I was involved with. I then can go to my family and personal life and give those areas my full attention.

Do you have any advice for nurses who might want to pursue this type of nursing career?

Good interpersonal skills, critical thinking skills, and organizational ability are important in parish nursing as in many other nursing careers.

Patient Education Coordinator

1. **Basic description**—The patient education coordinator is responsible for educating patients about their disease, medications, and all aspects of care needed following hospitalization or a clinic visit. Patient education is intended to help patients and families cope with a crisis, gather information, learn self-care, and use attitudes and strategies to promote optimal health. Patients who are well informed about their own health actively participate in their own health care decisions, are more likely to have better health overall and enjoy a better quality of life, have fewer illness-related complications, tend to be more compliant with medication and treatment regimens, and are less likely to be a drain on diminishing health care resources. Opportunities are available to work in hospitals, clinics, schools, health care organizations, and home health agencies.

2. **Educational requirements**—RN preparation with BSN; a MSN is preferred in most settings.

3. **Core competencies/skills needed:**
   - Ability to teach and inspire others
   - Maturity and dependability
   - Excellent communication skills
   - Ability to work with interdisciplinary teams
   - Interest in teaching patients and be knowledgeable about pathophysiology and health promotion
   - Teaching patients to manage acute and chronic illness
   - Postoperative teaching
   - Planning health education programs
   - Preparation of teaching materials

- Development of patient teaching plans in a form that is readily understood by the patient and pertinent to their unique circumstances
4. **Compensation**—Varies according to place of employment and geographic location.
5. **Employment outlook**—Moderate
6. **Related Web sites and professional organizations:**
   - Health Care Education Association: www.hcea-info.org/
   - National Council on Patient Information and Education: www.talkaboutrx.org/
   - Association of Community Health Nursing Educators: www.uncc.edu/achne/
   - United States Department of Health and Human Services: www.hhs.gov/

Peace Corps Volunteer

1. **Basic description**—Peace Corps volunteer nurses are assigned to specific jobs in third world countries. The history of the Peace Corps is the story of tens of thousands of people who have served as volunteers since 1961. Their individual experiences have composed a legacy of service that has become part of American history. There is a 27-month commitment. These health volunteers work in both rural and urban settings where they raise awareness about the need for health education and infrastructures for healthy environments. They work on a variety of health activities in the community, from educating and training in the areas of maternal/child health, basic nutrition, sanitation, oral rehydration therapy, and STDs/AIDS to organizing fund-raisers and community groups to obtain needed health care materials. Volunteers construct wells, tap springs, build latrines, and im-

prove potable water storage facilities and train local leaders to maintain water and sanitation systems and continue health programs after the volunteer departs. They teach in classrooms and model methodologies for teachers in local schools, undertake knowledge, attitude, and practice (KAP) surveys; assist clinics and/or ministerial planning offices in pinpointing health needs; devise educational projects to address prevailing health conditions; assist in the marketing of messages aimed at improving local health practices; carry out epidemiological studies.

2. **Educational requirements**—RN preparation.

3. **Core competencies/skills needed:**
    - Flexibility
    - Patience
    - Maturity
    - Curiosity
    - Enthusiasm for helping people
    - Dedication
    - Compassion
    - An understanding of different cultures
    - Desire to make a difference in a developing country
    - Excellent clinical skills

4. **Compensation**—Stipend.

5. **Employment outlook**—High

6. **Related Web site and professional organization:**
    - Peace Corps: www.peacecorps.gov

Pediatric Nurse Practitioner

1. **Basic description**—Pediatric nurse practitioners (PNP) are advanced practice nurses who provide management of care for

acutely and/or chronically ill pediatric patients. Hospitalization is frightening for a child, so the pediatric nurse specialist must know how to alleviate or assist in alleviating fears of children and their families. Children of a young age are often unable to express their emotions; therefore, it is the responsibility of the pediatric nurse specialist to be alert and aware of unexpressed needs. Work settings include acute care settings, subacute care settings, long-term care facilities, home care agencies, HMOs, ambulatory care settings, and schools.

2. **Educational requirements**—BSN, advanced practice licensure, MSN in pediatrics or family health, and PALS certification. Also requires continuing education for maintenance of licensure.

3. **Core competencies/skills needed:**
   - Special knowledge of growth and development
   - Knowledge of pediatric illnesses and their treatment
   - Ability to function independently
   - Ability to work with children and their families
   - Ability to set priorities and work independently
   - Collaboration with other health care providers

4. **Compensation**—Varies according to place of employment and geographic location.

5. **Employment outlook**—High

6. **Related Web sites and professional organizations:**
   - National Association of Pediatric Nurse Practitioners: www.napnap.org
   - Association of Pediatric Oncology Nurses (APON): www.apon.org
   - The National Certification Board of Pediatric Nurse Practitioners and Nurses: www.pnpcert.org
   - Society of Pediatric Nurses (SPN): www.pedsnurses.org

Perianesthesia Nurse

1. **Basic description**—Perianesthesia nursing provides intensive care to patients as they awake from anesthesia. The perianesthesia nurse prepares patients for the surgical experience, monitors and supports safe transition from anesthetized state to responsiveness, and readies patients for discharge from the perianesthesia care unit. Opportunities to work in perianesthesia care units in inpatient and outpatient settings, including freestanding operative settings, hospitals, and clinics.

2. **Educational requirements**—RN preparation. Certification is available. There are two certification programs for qualified registered nurses: the CPAN program (certified post anesthesia nurse) and the CAPA program (certified ambulatory perianesthesia nurse).

3. **Core competencies/skills needed:**
    *   Experience in medical-surgical and critical-care nursing
    *   Hands-on skills such as line placement, tube insertions, dressing changes, IV therapy, and positioning
    *   Flexibility
    *   Good assessment and decision-making skills
    *   Good management skills
    *   Technological ability
    *   Ability to teach
    *   Good interpersonal skills
    *   Must be able to respond to possible complications of anesthesia, including respiratory compromise, hypotension, emergence excitement, nausea and/or vomiting, pain
    *   Must be flexible and have an ability to manage stress

4. **Compensation**—Varies according to place of employment and geographic location.

5. **Employment outlook**—High
6. **Related Web sites and professional organizations:**
   - American Society of PeriAnesthesia Nurses (ASPAN): www.aspan.org
   - American Board of Perianesthesia Nursing Certification, Inc. (ABPANC): www.cpancapa.org/

Perinatal Nurse

1. **Basic description**—A perinatal nurse cares for women, infants, and their families from the onset of pregnancy through the 1st month of the newborn's life (perinatal period). The perinatal nurse needs to convey to the provider the patient's physiological status (vital signs, contractions, physical examination findings) and the well-being of the fetus as evidenced by fetal heart auscultation or monitoring in clear language. Perinatal nurses have opportunities to work in hospitals including specialty hospitals, health departments, medical offices, HMOs, clinics, birthing centers, nurse midwife practices, and home health agencies.

2. **Educational requirements**—RN preparation. Certification in perinatal nursing is available.

3. **Core competencies/skills needed:**
   - Interpersonal skills
   - Commitment
   - Oral and written communication skills
   - Ability to monitor the pregnancy
   - Ability to assess the progression of labor and maintain a sense of calm and comfort during labor
   - Ability to monitor the status of mother and baby
   - Knowledge of family support

- Skill in fostering the new mother-infant relationship and teach parenting skills
- Ability to assess and support the mother in her recovery from childbirth as well as evaluate the newborn's early adjustment to life

4. **Compensation**—Varies according to place of employment and geographic location.

5. **Employment outlook**—Moderate

6. **Related Web sites and professional organizations:**
   - Association of Women's Health, Obstetric and Neonatal Nurses: www.awhonn.org/
   - National Association of Neonatal Nurses (NANN): www.nann.org/
   - American Nurses Credentialing Center: www.nursingworld.org/ancc/

Pharmaceutical Representative

1. **Basic description**—RN involved in promoting and selling products from pharmaceutical companies. Practice settings include pharmaceutical companies and telemarketing companies.

2. **Educational requirements**—RN preparation; some companies prefer BSN.

3. **Core competencies/skills needed:**
   - Knowledge of product being promoted
   - Ability to manage time effectively
   - Good organizational skills
   - Marketing skills
   - Professional demeanor
   - Outgoing personality

- Good communication skills
- Self-motivated
- Ability to be flexible and travel

4. **Compensation**—Varies according to place of employment and geographic location.

5. **Employment outlook**—High

6. **Related Web sites and professional organizations:**

   - Industry managers and recruiters provide credible advice on the Who, What, When, Where, Why, and How of breaking into pharmaceutical sales: www.pharmaceutical-sales-info.com/ (there is a $15 fee to register on this website)
   - Pharmaceutical Representative Online: www.pharmrep.com/

Plastic and Reconstructive Surgery Nurse

1. **Basic description**—Plastic and reconstructive surgical nurses care for patients undergoing cosmetic surgery to correct aesthetic problems (e.g., face lift, breast augmentation), or to reconstruct some part of the body from disease, accident or malformations (e.g., skin lesions and tumors, congenital deformities, facial fractures, burns, ulcers, varicose veins, reconstruction after cancer surgery). There is often a great deal of patient happiness and appreciation following the surgery. Opportunities exist to work in hospitals, ambulatory surgery centers, and office practices.

2. **Educational requirements**—RN preparation. Certification is available as a certified plastic surgical nurse (CPSN) through the Plastic Surgical Nursing Certification Board, Inc.

3.   **Core competencies/skills needed:**
     *   Skills in patient care
     *   Specialized teaching about the patient's particular operative procedure
     *   Perioperative and postoperative care
     *   Excellent communication skills
     *   Consideration of clients' needs
4.   **Compensation**—Varies according to place of employment and geographic location.
5.   **Employment outlook**—Moderate
6.   **Related Web sites and professional organizations:**
     *   The American Society of Plastic and Reconstructive Surgical Nurses: www.karpinskimd.com/ASPRSN.html
     *   American Society of Plastic Surgical Nurses (ASPSN): www.aspsn.org/

Politician

1.   **Basic description**—A nurse politician is a nurse who is elected to public office. Nurse politicians serve in a variety of settings such as U.S. Congress, state government, boards of education, and nursing organizations. Given that there are more than 2.4 million nurses in this country, and that 1 in every 17 woman voters is a nurse, this represents an important growth area for nursing influence. There are currently two U.S. Congresswomen who are nurses: Rep. Lois Capps from California's 22nd district and Rep. Carolyn McCarthy from New York's 4th district.
2.   **Educational requirements**—RN preparation. Education and/ or experience in the area of political action.
3.   **Core competencies/skills needed:**
     *   Conviction to fight for your beliefs
     *   Interest in political and social issues

- Ability to be a decision maker
- Leadership ability
- Ability to identify a problem and develop a position and a plan to address the problem
- Ability to identify and articulate health care issues
- Skills in advocating for change
- Collaborating with other members of political team
- Designing legislation
- Experience in working for reforms in health care, education, and other identified areas of need

4. **Compensation**—Varies according to political position held and geographic location.

5. **Employment outlook**—Moderate

6. **Related Web sites and professional organizations:**

- American Nurses Association: www.ana.org
- The U.S. Congress: www.congress.gov

Private Duty Nurse

1. **Basic description**—Private duty nurses provide total individual patient care in the home or hospital environment with payment coming from a private source or insurance. Private duty nurses can work through an agency or independently.

2. **Educational requirements**—RN preparation.

3. **Core competencies/skills needed**—because the work is autonomous it is essential that they have the following competencies:

- Solid foundation in nursing skills
- Ability to assist patients with personal hygiene, activities of daily living, medication management, dressing changes, and intravenous therapy

- Ability to conduct complete assessments and monitoring when necessary
- Provide emotional support
- Problem-solving skills

4. **Compensation**—Varies according to place of employment and geographic location.

5. **Employment outlook**—Moderate

6. **Related Web site and professional organization:**

- No Web sites available.

Psychiatric Nurse

1. **Basic description**—Psychiatric nursing is centered around meeting the health needs of patients, with a particular focus on mental health. Psychiatric nurses may work with patients in an inpatient hospital setting, or a range of outpatient and community-based health care settings. A psychiatric nurse uses therapeutic communication to help patients of all ages better understand themselves and make behavior changes. Patients who are seen by psychiatric nurses may have a variety of illnesses, such as psychoses, personality, and mood disorders, substance abuse disorders, and depression, just to name a few. Psychiatric nurses may work with child, adolescent, or adult patients. Psychiatric nursing involves understanding not only the mental, but the biological aspects of human thought processes and behaviors as well. Pharmacology also plays a role in psychiatric nursing, because there are many different medications used to treat mental illness and nurses must understand the physiological effects of these medications. Psychiatric nurses may be prepared as advanced practice nurses and as psychotherapists.

2. **Educational requirements** — RN preparation. Past work experience in any setting where there was a focus on therapeutic communication is extremely important. A solid medical-surgical background with strong assessment experience is important in order to understand and recognize the physiologic effects of psychiatric treatment. Certification is available as a psychiatric/ mental health nurse, clinical specialist, or nurse practitioner through the American Nurses Credentialing Center; psychiatric nurses may be licensed as individual, family, or group therapists.

3. **Core competencies/skills needed:**
    - Excellent communication skills, because therapeutic communication is used in every encounter with patients.
    - Strong critical thinking skills
    - Ability to work with child, adolescent, adult, and elderly patients
    - Observation skills to recognize and understand a patient's nonverbal communication
    - Excellent crisis management skills in order to handle potentially dangerous situations and protect themselves and their parents from harm
    - Ability to deal with patients who may be uncooperative or even dangerous at times
    - Ability to treat patients with a holistic, nonjudgmental attitude
    - Values for mental health as an important aspect of the health care system
    - Patient advocacy skills

4. **Compensation** — Varies according to place of employment and geographic location.

5. **Employment outlook** — High

6. **Related Web sites and professional organizations:**
    - American Psychiatric Nurses Association: www.apna.org
    - Alliance for Psychosocial Nursing: www.psychnurse.org/
    - American Nurses Credentialing Center: www.nursingworld.org/ancc/index.htm
    - Association of Child and Adolescent Psychiatric Nurses (ACAPN): www.ispn-psych.org/html/acapn.html

Public and Community Health Nurse

1. **Basic description** — Public health nurses and community health nurses provide individual and population-focused community-oriented care. Community nurses participate in assessing the population in order to determine needed health services with the goal to improve the overall health of the community through disease prevention, health promotion, and wellness/health education. The public health nurse's goal in general is to promote and protect the health of populations using social and public health, public health sciences, and knowledge from nursing. They may also be involved in community health fairs, educational events, and establishing relationships with community organizations. They often assume responsibility for personnel, resources, and patient care in public health and will develop, implement, and evaluate educational programs and activities designed to meet these needs. They may also be involved in one-on-one education, making follow-up phone calls, and conducting home visits, with appropriate documentation of these services. This person may also establish and control the budget and support standards of nursing in the public health practice.

2. **Educational requirements** — RN preparation. Certification as a community health nurse and as a clinical specialist in community health nursing is available through the American Nurses Credentialing Center.

3. **Core competencies/skills needed:**
   - Knowledge of public health and epidemiology
   - Collaborative abilities and team skills

- Assertiveness and self-reliance
- Interpersonal skills
- Analytic skills
- Policy development skills
- Cultural competency
- Management skills
- Must enjoy team effort and providing service in the community

4. **Compensation**—Varies according to place of employment and geographic location.
5. **Employment outlook**—High
6. **Related Web site and professional organization:**
   - American Public Health Association: www.apha.org

Pulmonary/Respiratory Nurse

1. **Basic description**—A pulmonary and respiratory nurse promotes pulmonary health for individuals, families, and communities, and cares for persons with pulmonary dysfunction throughout the lifespan. Respiratory nursing may be preventive, acute, critical, or rehabilitative. There are opportunities to work in hospitals, extended care centers, private companies, health departments, office practices, and clinics.
2. **Educational requirements**—RN preparation.
3. **Core competencies/skills needed:**
   - Knowledge of respiratory disease such as, asthma, chronic obstructive pulmonary disease (COPD), TB, cystic fibrosis, and respiratory failure
   - Excellent patient and family relationships and teaching abilities

- Team skills to work with other members of the health care team
- Ability to deal with issues of grief and loss
- Strong assessment skills
- Knowledge of oxygen therapies, assisted ventilation, and suctioning
- Patience for patient non-adherence to regimen and tobacco abuse
- Ability to discuss smoking cessation techniques, ability to administer and teach pharmacologic interventions

4. **Compensation**—Varies according to place of employment and geographic location.

5. **Employment outlook**—Moderate

6. **Related Web sites and professional organizations:**
   - Respiratory Nursing Society (RNS): www.respiratorynursingsociety.org
   - American Association of Cardiovascular and Pulmonary Rehabilitation: www.aacvpr.org

---

Quality Assurance Nurse

1. **Basic description**—Nurses in quality assurance (QA) promote quality, cost-effective outcomes for an organization by interpreting and applying policies and procedures guidelines. They must identify and coordinate the needs of the patients with needs of the provider and orchestrate patient care among multiple caregivers through the continuum from pre-admission through discharge based on age, cultural, and individual patient needs. These nurses support and act as liaisons with the payers, providers, and patients and serve as the primary patient information resource for payers. QA nurses collaborate with physicians and

treatment teams to develop patient care guidelines and serves on quality improvement teams. There are QA opportunities to work in the private sector, hospitals, and government facilities.

2. **Educational requirements**—RN preparation; BSN preferred.

3. **Core competencies/skills needed:**
   - Training or experience in utilization review, discharge planning, and case management
   - Strong interpersonal and communication skills
   - Acute care skills
   - Ability to identify problems such as under or over utilization of services
   - Self directed with positive attitude
   - Ability to promote and maintain quality care through analysis

4. **Compensation**—Varies according to place of employment and geographic location.

5. **Employment outlook**—High

6. **Related Web sites and professional organizations:**
   - Agency for Healthcare Research Quality: www.ahrq.gov
   - Joint Commission for Accreditation of Health Care Organizations: www.jcaho.org

Radiology Nurse

1. **Basic description**—A nurse working primarily in the hospital setting, assisting, performing, and teaching in the role of radiological imaging. Contemporary radiology departments are equipped with state-of-the-art imaging capacities and radiology nurses assist in the care of patients undergoing invasive procedures.

2. **Educational requirements**—RN preparation.

3. **Core competencies/skills needed:**
   - Strong anatomy and physiology theory base and education in disease processes of human body
   - Technical proficiency and knowledge of procedures to be performed
   - Good teaching skills to prepare and help clients reach best outcome from a test/procedure
   - Knowledge of good body mechanics for optimal positioning of patient for procedure
   - Ability to interpret and identify life-threatening arrhythmias
   - Skill in reviewing patient's clinical history for potential indicators that might contraindicate the procedure
   - Advocating for patient safety
4. **Compensation**—Varies according to place of employment and geographic location.
5. **Employment outlook**—Moderate
6. **Related Web site and professional organization:**
   - Radiological Society of North American, Inc.: www.rsna.org

Recruiter

1. **Basic description**—Nurse recruiters develop and implement short- and long-term recruitment plans and strategies to meet nurse staffing needs. They also create, coordinate, and maintain a wide range of cost-effective recruitment strategies to generate applicant pools and hires. Work settings include hospitals, nursing homes, schools of nursing, and travel health care companies.
2. **Educational requirements**—RN preparation.
3. **Core competencies/skills needed:**
   - Excellent interpersonal skills
   - Ability to screen and interview prospective job applicants

- Ability to develop relationships with the various nursing programs/schools in the area to promote nursing career opportunities and market
- Contacts, interviews, and places nurses in jobs at a health care facility
- Self-directed and self-motivated
- Team skills
- Marketing skills
- Excellent phone voice, positive and enthusiastic
- Organizational skills
- Focus with attention to detail

4. **Compensation**—Varies according to place of employment and geographic location.
5. **Employment outlook**—Moderate
6. **Related Web sites and professional organizations:**
   - National Association for Health Care Recruitment: www.nahcr.com/
   - Nurse Recruiter for Nurses by Nurses: www.nurse-recruiter.com

---

Rehabilitation Nurse

1. **Basic description**—Rehabilitation nursing is a specialty practice area that involves care of individuals with altered functional ability and altered lifestyle. Rehabilitation nurses begin to work with individuals and their families soon after a disabling injury or chronic illness strikes, and they continue to provide support after these individuals go home or return to work or school. The goal of rehabilitation nursing is to assist individuals with disabilities and chronic illness in the restoration, maintenance, and promotion of optimal health. Rehabilitation nursing practice

occurs in many settings and involves a variety of roles. Most opportunities exist in hospitals (including specialty hospitals), long-term care facilities, and free-standing facilities.

2. **Educational requirements**—RN preparation. A registered nurse with at least 2 years of practice in rehabilitation nursing can earn distinction as a Certified Rehabilitation Registered Nurse (CRRN) by successfully completing an examination that validates expertise. Likewise, a registered nurse with a CRRN and a master's degree or doctorate in nursing can earn certification as a Certified Rehabilitation Registered Nurse-Advanced (CRRN-A).

3. **Core competencies/skills needed:**
   - Long-term patient and colleague relationships
   - Ability to work with clients from infancy to elderly
   - Teamwork and collaboration
   - Patient and family education
   - Innovative thinking
   - Autonomy and independence
   - Skilled at treating alterations in functional ability and lifestyle resulting from injury, disability, and chronic illness
   - Skill in providing comfort, therapy, and education
   - Skill in promoting health-conducive adjustments, support adaptive capabilities, and promote achievable independence
   - Skill in promoting holistic, comprehensive, and compassionate end-of-life care, including promotion of comfort and relief of pain
   - Excellent functional assessment skills
   - Skill in team management as they act as a multisystem integrators and team leaders, working with physicians, therapists, and others to solve problems and promote patients' maximal independence
   - Ability to work with others to adapt ongoing care to the resources available distinguishes the practice of rehabilitation nursing
   - Goal-oriented and focused on returning patients to optimal functionality
   - Ability to provide holistic care to meet patients' medical, vocational, educational, environmental, and spiritual needs
   - Ability to function not only as caregivers but also as coordinators, collaborators, counselors, and case managers

4. **Compensation**—Varies according to place of employment and geographic location.
5. **Employment outlook**—Moderate
6. **Related Web site and professional organization:**
   - Association of Rehabilitation Nurses (ARN): www.rehabnurse.org/

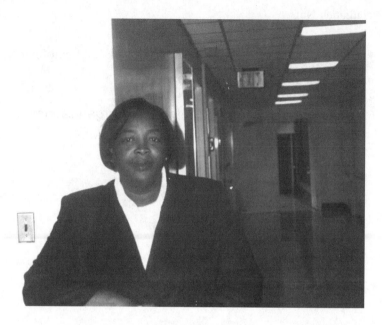

Betty Furr, Rehabilitation Nursing Administrator.

An Interview with
Betty Furr,
Rehabilitation Nursing
Administrator

What is your educational background in nursing (and other areas) and what formal credentials do you hold?

I received my associate of Applied Science degree in Nursing from Marymount University, then received a BSN from the same university. I have a master's degree in Nursing from Catholic University of America. I received a certificate in Hospital Administration from Howard University and a certificate in Risk Management from the Institute of Medical

Law and a certificate in Bioethics and Medical Humanities from NYU. I am currently a PhD student at NYU.

How did you first become interested in your current career?

I first became interested in rehabilitation nursing while working as adjunct faculty for a nursing program. I was a clinical instructor. My students received practical experience in fundamental nursing skills at one of the area subacute nursing and rehabilitation facilities (SNF). I was profoundly impacted by the experience of seeing the status of some of the patients' post-acute hospital care. I saw patients making good progress toward community re-entry. I saw the hope they had for returning to the life they once lived. Young and old held the belief that they could and would succeed in reaching their goal. I particularly recall a 29-year-old young man who had suffered multiple trauma from a motor vehicle accident. He had spent a number of months in the acute hospital prior to being transferred to the SNF. His road to recovery had been long and difficult, but his desire to get well and return to his family was firm. His perseverance was rewarded with his realizing his goal. There were many similar cases that made me enjoy working in rehabilitation nursing.

What are the most rewarding aspects of your career?

The most rewarding aspects of my career are my being a part of the passion and joy of dedicated, committed staff that give so much of themselves to very challenged patient populations and the feelings of accomplishment I realize from seeing so many good outcomes for our patients.

Describe a typical workday in your current job.

A typical workday in my role as director of a rehabilitation center might start with a meeting with the chairman of Rehabilitation Medicine, then clinical rounds in one of the patient services areas. For example: Out-Patients Services, Sports Therapy Center, Spinal Cord Injury Program In-Patient Services, Brain Injury Program In-Patient Services, or Medically Complex Rehabilitation In-Patient Services. Typically, I will have a standard coaching, supervision, counseling meeting with a member of the center leadership team, that is, one of the therapy managers or nursing managers or the admissions coordinator. I usually meet with one of the medical directors regarding anything from program management to funding. Or I might meet with one of the physiatrists, nurses, physical therapists, occupational therapists, psychologists, speech language pathologists, social workers, or dieticians regarding a clinical issue. I will attend a patient services/nursing or hospital executive leadership meeting or an executive or nursing clinical review committee meeting. I am usually also involved with a number of educational or performance improvement initiatives. Then I return to my office and answer e-mails, return phone calls, and so forth.

The rehabilitation center serves as a core department for rehabilitation services medical center–wide. I often address issues relative to these services with attending physicians and other area directors or managers throughout the hospital.

What advice would you give to someone contemplating the same career path in nursing?

I would advise someone contemplating the same career path in nursing to explore the opportunities in rehabilitation nursing practice. Rehabilitation nursing occurs in a variety of settings and encompasses the full scope of health care from primary prevention to community re-entry and life-care planning. The patient's needs represent a wide range of health management issues—for example, neurologic, pulmonary, cardiac, musculoskeletal, obstetrical, GYN, GU, GI, and endocrine. The ages of the patients are from new born to the oldest old. (My oldest patient up to this point was 104 years of age.) Rehabilitation nursing practice is broad enough to allow the choice of a career path that speaks to ones specific passion within the professional practice of nursing.

How do you balance career and other aspects of your life?

I try to balance career and other aspects of my life by inclusion. I believe to live as a whole person I must incorporate successful approaches to addressing the needs of mind, body, and spirit. Therefore, I pursue experiences that allow this. To enhance my mind's activity I have continued my formal education.

To address the needs of the body, I have engaged in numerous physical training programs. I recently started to work with a personal trainer to assist in my efforts to bring greater balance to the body.

To nurture my spirit I engage in daily spiritual activities. I practice meditation. I attend church. I travel to other parts of the world to learn and better understand other cultures and to increase my love and appreciation for my fellow man. I have studied various traditional approaches to spirituality. I am participating in a 4-year program of study of Hawaiian spirituality and myth.

I find the time to enjoy all aspects of my life, my family, friends, and others.

Do you have any other advice for other nurses who might want to pursue this type of nursing career?

The only other advice I have for other nurses who might want to pursue rehabilitation nursing as a career is to actively consider this career path. It allows for traditional as well as non-traditional nurse roles, from direct hands-on-care to corporate style leadership as a director of a center or institute. There are opportunities within this career path that might enhance or reinvigorate your love of nursing.

Researcher

1. **Basic description**—A nurse researcher conducts studies related to individual, family and community health, symptoms of illness, nursing interventions to promote health and decrease incidence or symptoms of illness, and research related to nursing and health care delivery including workforce planning. The research may involve a large project funded through the National Institutes of Health or a small project supported by funds from the researcher's institution. Research requires an attention to detail; thus, the work is methodical and sometimes tedious. Researchers may work alone or in teams with other nurse researchers or clinicians; often the research undertaken by nurse scientists is multidisciplinary in nature, thus requiring the researchers to engage in team building and team functioning. Researchers often work under great time pressure to meet deadlines for funding agencies, or publication deadlines.

2. **Educational requirements**—PhD degree in nursing or related discipline.

3. **Core competencies/skills needed:**
    *   Research methods knowledge and skills
    *   Knowledge of statistical methods and analyses
    *   Grant writing skills
    *   Analytical and organizational skills
    *   Writing skills
    *   Team building skills are often required

4. **Compensation**—Varies according to place of employment and geographic location.

5. **Employment outlook**—High

6. **Related Web sites and professional organizations:**
   - National Institute of Nursing Research; a branch of the U.S. Health and Human Services National Institutes of Health: www.nih.gov/ninr/
   - Sigma Theta Tau International: www.nursingsociety.com

Risk-Management Nurse

1. **Basic description**—Risk-management nurses have special knowledge and interest in the work environment of nurses and the injuries nurses sustain as a result of environmental exposures. They may be consultants responsible for reviewing medical records, policies, and procedures, and thus would be aware of legal aspects and their implications. Risk-management nurses conduct programs covering aspects of documentation and internal procedures in order to protect patients and staff from injuries.

2. **Educational requirements**—RN preparation.

3. **Core competencies/skills needed:**
   - Ability to view every environment as a whole, by an objective observer in relation to patient and nurse safety
   - Computer skills
   - Analytical skills
   - Communication skills
   - Handle multiple tasks simultaneously
   - Sharp visual acuity
   - Keen judgement
   - Excellent observational skills
   - Strong assessment skills

4. **Compensation**—Varies according to place of employment and geographic location.

5. **Employment outlook**—High

6. **Related Web sites and professional organizations:**
   - Agency for Health Care Research Quality: www.ahrq.gov
   - Joint Commission for Accreditation of Health Care Organizations: www.jcaho.org
   - American Nurses Association: www.ana.org

Rural Health Nurse

1. **Basic description**—A rural health nurse is a generalist who practices professional nursing in communities with relatively low populations that are geographically and often culturally isolated. Rural nurses have close ties to and interaction with the communities in which they practice, and often practice with a great deal of autonomy and independence. A commitment to providing care at the individual, family, and community level is central to the role of a rural nurse. A strong and varied experience base is crucial in rural nursing, as the population that the rural nurse must care for ranges from infants to the elderly. Therefore, a rural nurse must know everything about every stage of life. Experience with rural communities is also a benefit in order to understand the cultural context within which the people live. For most rural nurses, traveling between isolated communities is part of their role. Rural nurses may operate from a clinic or small hospital, while others may base themselves out of a large mobile health center. The activities by rural nurses are vast; a nurse may give prenatal care to a 25-year-old woman and then treat an 80-year-old for a bladder infection, or teach a recent stroke victim how to get in and out of the shower.

2. **Educational requirements**—RN preparation.

3. **Core competencies/skills needed:**
   - Physical assessment and emergency/trauma management skills are vital to the practice or a rural nurse

- Skilled in all areas of nursing, with clinical and assessment skills that reflect this proficiency
- Critical care skills
- An aptitude for teaching
- A wide knowledge of resources within the community
- Management skills
- Surgical, obstetric, IV therapy skills and the ability to operate and troubleshoot equipment are other useful skills to possess
- Knowledgeable about areas such as pharmacy, the region in which one is practicing, as well as an in-depth awareness of cultural norms and values
- Ability to adapt to the resources that are available
- Ability to use innovative and creative solutions to the challenges that exist in locations without major medical centers
- Ability to practice independently and even without the supplies and equipment available that one needs
- Value the close interaction they have with the individuals, families, and communities they serve

4. **Compensation**—Varies according to place of employment and geographic location.
5. **Employment outlook**—Moderate
6. **Related Web site and professional organization:**
   - Rural Nursing Organization: www.rno.org

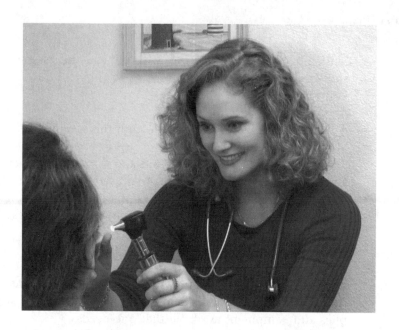

Maria Humphry, Rural Health Nurse.

An Interview with
Maria Humphry,
Rural Health Nurse

What is your educational background in nursing (and other areas) and what formal credentials do you hold?

My credentials are as follows: I expect to receive my PhD in Nursing in 2005, from Loyola University. I have an MSN in Nursing, Pediatric Nurse Practitioner, from Case Western Reserve University. I have a BSN in Nursing, with a Psychology minor from Dominican College.

My certifications include sexual assault nurse examiner, parish nurse, prescriptive authority, drug enforcement agency license, community health nurse, registered nurse, public health nurse.

I started out as a certified nurse's aide and worked as an obstetrics nurse/neonatal intensive care nurse before becoming a pediatric nurse practitioner. I taught at the University of Montana and currently hold the position of adjunct assistant professor at Montana State University College of Nursing. I serve on many nursing committees and am involved in many public services in my community.

How did you first become interested in your current career?

I first became interested in nursing as a young child. My father is a pediatrician and my mother is a nurse. I can remember numerous hours I spent going on rounds with my father at the local hospitals on Saturday mornings. I remember vividly how I admired the nurses and their role in caring for the babies in the nursery. This is when I decided I wanted to work in the medical field. I originally wanted to be a physician; however, after my first semester in college I realized I liked the act of caring much more than the act or curing, therefore I changed to nursing. After my undergraduate education I realized that I enjoyed caring for patients but I wanted more independence and autonomy in my work. This is when I decided to become a nurse practitioner.

What are the most rewarding aspects of your career?

As a nurse practitioner the absolute most rewarding aspect of my career is seeing the patients who I have cared for in the worst of situations recover and lead healthy lives. I like walking into an exam room knowing that parents depend upon my judgment, skill, and decision making. I enjoy being helpful, answering concerned questions, and giving hope when it is needed.

As a university professor I enjoy watching the "firsts" with my students. Times like the first injection, first catheter, or even the first medication administration are all very stressful events in nursing student's lives. When a student looks up after successfully completing a first task and smiles, I know my job is worth every effort of energy I give it. To experience the successes of my students no matter how small makes my job rewarding.

Describe a typical workday in your current position.

A typical workday as a nurse practitioner starts at 7:00 A.M. I try to leave my home by 7:40 to make the 1 hour and 20 minute drive down the Bitterroot valley to the rural town of Hamilton, Montana, where my practice is located. I generally start seeing patients at 9:00 A.M. I see patients every half hour until noon. Most of the time I see typical childhood ailments (ear infections, strep throat, asthma). I have a 1-hour lunch then it is back to seeing patients until 5:00 P.M. A typical day usually has one or two difficult diagnoses or acutely ill children. It is not uncommon for me to stay late waiting upon lab results or to have an x-ray read over at the hospital. Once all my phone calls are returned to concerned parents, all the prescription refills are made and my patient chart notes are done I head for home around 6:00 or 7:00 P.M. The drive home is usually long and I am very tired. When I look back, however, it was worth every minute of my time.

What advice would you give to someone contemplating the same career path in nursing?

I would encourage a student to do several things when looking at nursing as a career. First he or she needs to decide what they want to do for a career. Do they want to make money right away to support a family? Do they want to work in floor nursing and maybe become a unit manager some day? Or, do they want to become the nursing supervisor for a hospital or run a home health agency? Depending upon the student's career goals I would recommend a LPN, RN, or BSN program. Those that want to have the most flexibility and options to expand their talents will definitely want to become BSNs. Those who are considering becoming rural nurse practitioners like myself I encourage them to find a mentor. I used several mentors both were pediatricians who working in rural medicine and held many of the same values and ethics for treating patients as myself. It is important to find someone to take you under his or her wing and guide you. Rural nursing is independent, and the support of another who has walked the same path is essential. There will be many times when your mentor is called upon to assist in a difficult situation or decision; having the consultation and support is important.

How do you balance career and other aspects of your life?

There is a very delicate balance between nursing and my personal life. I, like so many in my field, can become consumed with caring for others. I always remind myself that I must take personal time out for myself in order to serve those I care for in the best fashion possible. The diversity I hold with teaching 4 days a week and private practice 1 day a week is a nice balance. I enjoy the university setting with its learning atmosphere and innovative energy. I also look forward to returning to my little patients at my practice 1 day a week. Crawling around on the floor and making faces with my patients is what pediatric nursing is all about! I always make time to work out and plan frequent weekend trips away from work. I find that it is difficult at times since nursing is such a natural part of my being, however, I know that a good nurse is one who can take care of him or herself as well as the patient.

Do you have any advice for nurses who might want to pursue this type of nursing career?

For those men and women who know they want to become nurse practitioners I would encourage them to do so in a timely fashion. Many programs today recognize the professional world of the Nurse Practitioner and understand its uniqueness. No longer are programs requiring one or more years experience as a nurse before applying to graduate school to become a nurse practitioner. I tell my students "does experience help? Sure it does. Is it necessary to make a great Nurse Practitioner? No" If a nurse wants to further his/her career why stop half way? It is time we as a profession stopped using double standards. Pre medical students don't stop their career plans to get some hospital experience before heading to medical school, why should nurses?

School Nurse

1. **Basic description**—The school nurse practices professional nursing within an educational setting with the goal of assisting students to develop to their greatest physical, emotional, and intellectual ability. School nurses promote health and safety practices and provide interventions to actual and potential health problems. These nurses respond to acute injuries within the school population, as well as assist students to manage chronic conditions, such as food allergies, asthma, and other illnesses. Practice settings include school systems, state health departments, and county health departments.

2. **Educational requirements**—RN preparation. Some school systems and/or health departments are requiring that school nurses have baccalaureate or masters degrees in nursing. For example, the State of Massachusetts requires a minimum of 2 full years as a nurse in a child, community health, or other relevant clinical nursing setting.

3. **Core competencies/skills needed:**
    *   General experience with children
    *   Strong foundation in physical assessment and first aid and emergency care
    *   A solid skill base and understanding of pediatric medicine
    *   Knowledge of developmental stages is very important in order to provide age appropriate care
    *   Strong communication and interpersonal skills to assess and determine the health care needs of the children and their families
    *   Computer skills to chart and track students' records and immunization status

- Ability to relate to children and communicate patients and the school community
- Ability to provide health education
- Responsible for medication management of children while they are in school
- Skills to participate as a member of a multidisciplinary education team and collaborate with other members of the educational environment
- Ability to provide care for minor ailments such as a scraped knee as well as potentially serious conditions such as an allergic reaction or a major injury
- Ensure the safety and well-being of all the children in the school
- Ability to deal with issues such as school violence, suicide, and unwanted teen pregnancies

4. **Compensation**—Varies according to place of employment and geographic location

5. **Employment outlook**—Moderate

6. **Related Web sites and professional organizations:**
   - National Association of School Nurses (NASN): www.nasn.org
   - The Association of School Nurses of Connecticut: http://schoolnurse.vservers.com/
   - National Association of State School Nurse Consultants

Space Nurse/Astronaut

1. **Basic description**—Space nurses provide on-the-ground monitoring and a full range of health services to more than 400 astronauts, who are screened to determine if they meet NASA health requirements and, in some cases, military stipulations.

These data must be meticulously documented, because they are used to follow the health of astronauts throughout their lifetimes and to determine service eligibility, and are crucial to mission safety. A dispensary staffed by nurses is included in NASA's long-term plans, which call for larger space stations and a permanent lunar base. Flight Medicine Clinic (FMC) nurses also coordinate dietary and fitness services; clinic nurses staff a "sick call" service for astronauts to use before and after flight. At the first sign of physical discomfort, an astronaut first contacts a nurse, who administers appropriate treatment. Other nurses are employed as support staff for proctology and cardiovascular clinics and as instructors in the basis of self-assessment and medication administration for astronauts. Space Nurse Society (SNS) members now meet at yearly conferences to exchange ideas, share research findings, and discuss the application of nursing methods used on Earth in space settings. Many members are nurse researchers who study the health risks associated with space travel.

2. **Educational requirements**—RN preparation; graduate preparation required for researchers.

3. **Core competencies/skills needed:**
   - Excellent assessment skills
   - Interest in and knowledge of aerospace industry and challenges
   - Mental health skills
   - Innovation and creativity
   - Knowledge of physics and engineering

4. **Compensation**—Varies.

5. **Employment outlook**—Currently, space nurses are not eligible for onboard service in the astronaut program. The number of "flight nurses" working directly with flight crews is small but opportunities can be expected to increase significantly over the next two decades. Nurses who earn additional credentials in physics or engineering may one day join a space team.

6. **Related Web sites and professional organizations:**
   - The Space Nursing Society (SNS): www.geocities.com/spacenursingsociety/
   - The Mars Society: www.marssociety.org

- The National Aeronautics and Space Administration (NASA) Headquarters: www.nasa.gov
- NASA jobs: www.nasajobs.nasa.gov

Spinal Cord Injury Nurse

1. **Basic description**—Spinal cord injury (SCI) nurses play a vital role in maintaining the patient's respiratory, gastrointestinal, urinary, musculoskeletal, and integumentary systems and in providing psychological support to the patient and family. Caring for a patient with a spinal cord injury is complex and demanding. Although the primary focus in acute care management is directed toward sustaining life, it is critical that nurses involved in acute care management realize the effect their care has on the patient's rehabilitation and future life. By working to avoid preventable complications that cause additional morbidity and delay rehabilitation, nurses in acute care settings can help people with this devastating injury have the best possible opportunity to regain their health.

2. **Educational requirements**—RN preparation.

3. **Core competencies/skills needed:**
   - Excellent clinical skills
   - Team skills for collaboration with respiratory and physical therapy to protect respiratory function
   - Knowledge of the rehabilitation processes used in provision of care
   - Good interpersonal skills
   - Skills in helping patients and families manage anxiety by providing them with accurate information about the consequences of the injury in terms they can understand and by offering realistic hope for the future

4. **Compensation**—Varies according to place of employment and geographic location.

5. **Employment outlook**—Moderate

6. **Related Web sites and professional organizations:**
   - American Spinal Injury Association (ASIA): www.asia-spinalinjury.org/index.html
   - Spinal Cord Injury: The acute phase (two-part series), by Maureen Habel, MA, RN: www.nurseweek.com/ce/ce107a.asp#ref

Staff Development Educator

1. **Basic description**—The staff development educator incorporates a variety of roles into the teaching of new staff members. They are responsible for the basic orientation and continuing education for new nurses and nursing staff employed by hospitals and other health care organizations. They monitor the overall staff compliance with clinical performance standards and participate in providing ongoing continuing education for nursing staff. They may specialize in certain clinical areas (e.g., gerontology, oncology, or may be generalists). These educators function in a number of settings including hospitals, senior centers, clinics, HMOs, and schools of nursing.

2. **Educational requirements**—RN preparation; BSN or MSN preferred in some settings.

3. **Core competencies/skills needed:**
   - Ability to set priorities
   - Knowledge of adult learning theory
   - Ability to be an effective teacher
   - Excellent communication skills
   - Commitment to life long learning

- Ability to develop and implement lesson plans
- Staff development experience
- Positive attitude and enthusiasm for learning
- Ability to manage time effectively
- Ability to function autonomously

4. **Compensation**—Varies according to place of employment and geographic setting.

5. **Employment outlook**—Moderate

6. **Related Web site and professional organization:**
   - National Nursing Staff Development Organization (NNSDO): www.nnsdo.org

---

Telemetry Nurse

1. **Basic description**—Telemetry nurses assess acute changes in patients and work in a fast-paced environment. These nurses monitor the heart rhythm of patients in special care units of hospitals and analyze heart rhythms, interpret ECGs, note arrhythmias, and intervene in emergency situations.

2. **Educational requirements**—RN preparation.

3. **Core competencies/skills needed:**
   - Excellent clinical skills
   - Critical thinking ability
   - Cardiovascular knowledge, including anatomy and physiology and cardiac disease processes
   - Skill in patient teaching about medications, dietary changes, and post-MI activity restrictions
   - Flexibility given the unpredictability of the patient status
   - Ability to use technology available for patient monitoring

4. **Compensation**—Varies according to place of employment and geographic location.

5. **Employment outlook**—Moderate
6. **Related Web site and professional organization:**
   • No Web sites available.

Telephone Triage Nurse

1. **Basic description**—A telephone triage nurse provides a variety of services and information to patients over the phone. Most often, they are using written protocols to guide their practice and are determining the urgency of care needed and scheduling appointments or directing callers to health care providers as needed. Accordingly, the goal of this unique form of nursing is to decrease unnecessary visits to physicians, nurse practitioners, and the emergency room as well as to provide information for self-care. Some triage nurses working for medical practices or clinics may be familiar with the patient and their health status. More often, though, the nurse must use his or her excellent communication and information gathering skills to determine the best course of action for the patient. Triage nurses deal with the entire spectrum, from healthy patients to the acute and chronically ill. Triage nurses usually have regular hours but there is not any direct patient contact and triage nurses may spend long hours at a desk on the telephone and computer. There are opportunities to work in a variety of settings such as medical offices, HMOs, insurance companies, hospitals, clinics, and triage centers.

2. **Educational requirements**—RN preparation.

3. **Core competencies/skills needed:**
   • Previous experience with triage, either on the telephone or in an emergency room
   • Critical thinking skills

- Ability to determine the problem within the first few sentences of a conversation; a certain intuitive ability can be useful in assessing the situation and making the correct decision for the patient
- Superior verbal communication skills are essential
- Strong assessment skills
- Excellent clinical skills
- Crisis intervention skills
- Typing and computer ability to keep track of information gathered in the telephone conversation
- Teaching ability, as patients may require instruction for self-care and/or symptom management
- Ability to remain calm in high stress situations

4. **Compensation**—Varies according to place of employment and geographic location.

5. **Employment outlook**—High

6. **Related Web sites and professional organizations:**
   - All Health Net: Telephone Triage Nursing: www.allhealthnet.com/Nursing/Telephone+Triage/
   - Information about Telephone Triage for Nurses: www.geocities.com/hanson1517/ NURSESINFORMATIONPAGE.html
   - International Telenurses Association: www.intellinurse.org

Transplant Nurse

1. **Basic description**—The transplant nurse cares for recipient and living-donor patients throughout the transplantation process from end-stage disease processes to the preoperative, operative, and postoperative care. The transplant nurse is most often employed by the hospital with a transplant center. Practice roles can

include nurse practitioner, case manager, transplant coordinator, research nurse, organ procurement nurse, and clinical specialist.

2. **Educational requirements**—RN preparation; BSN or MSN is often preferred.

3. **Core competencies/skills needed:**
   - Knowledge of transplant processes
   - Communication skills
   - Excellent communication skills
   - Teaching skills
   - Knowledge of high-tech treatments
   - Sensitivity in dealing with emotional and ethical issues
   - Technological skills
   - Ability to work with interdisciplinary team

4. **Compensation**—Varies according to place of employment and geographic location.

5. **Employment outlook**—High

6. **Related Web sites and professional organizations:**
   - International Transplant Nurses Society: www.itns.org/
   - International Society for Heart and Lung Transplantation: www.ishlt.org/

Travel Nurse

1. **Basic description**—Travel nurses are those who travel and take temporary nursing assignments, usually lasting 8 to 26 weeks (average is 13 weeks), in locations of the nurse's choice, in facilities across the United States and internationally. Travel nurses often work in hospital settings in staff nurse positions, but may also be found on cruise ships, in rural settings, or other roles that require the skill of a registered nurse. A travel nurse

works with an agency that makes arrangements for the position, provides accommodations at the location, and pays for travel expenses. The work activities depend on the location and type of the assignment. A nurse could go from a tertiary ICU caring for a postoperative coronary bypass patient to a small 30-bed hospital where nurses care for a child with pneumonia next to an elderly patient with a stroke. Travel nurses are those who thrive on diversity and enjoy the opportunity to travel and experience new places and cultures.

2. **Educational requirements**—RN preparation; experience as a nurse is often preferred but not required.

3. **Core competencies/skills needed:**
   - Strong clinical skills; a critical care background is highly recommended, but not required
   - Flexibility and adaptability
   - Strong communication skills and the ability to get along with people to help integration within a unit and foster positive working relationships
   - Adaptable to change

4. **Compensation**—Varies according to place of employment and geographic location.

5. **Employment outlook**—High

6. **Related Web sites and professional organizations:**
   - National Association of Traveling Nurses: www.travelingnurse.org
   - NursesRx: www.nursesrx.com
   - Preferred Healthcare Staffing: www.preferredhealthcare.com
   - TravelNursing.com: www.travelnurse.com
   - PSR Nurses: www.psrnurses.com

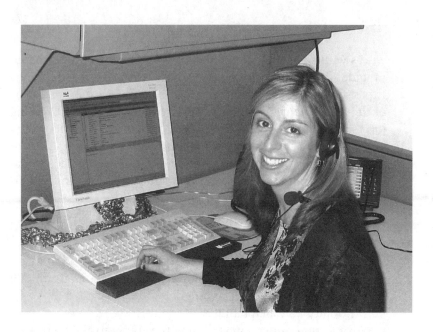

Lisa Hasnosi, Travel Nurse.

An Interview with
Lisa Hasnosi,
Travel Nurse

What is your educational background in nursing (and other areas) and what formal credentials do you hold?

My credentials are as follows: a BA in Psychology and Nutrition from Southern Connecticut State University and an ASN in Nursing from Ohlone College.

I worked as a rehabilitation activity leader and certified nursing assistant before becoming a registered nurse. I have worked in a variety of settings and positions, including medical clinics, large hospitals, as a clinical nurse supervisor, case manager, as a charge nurse on various psychiatric units, and as a consultant. My work currently is that of traveling nurse and RN coordinator. I travel both domestically and internationally.

How did you first become interested in your current career?

After I received my bachelor of arts degree in psychology, I started working at Yale Psychiatric Institute as a mental health counselor. I thought I wanted to become a psychologist, but after working with nurses, I found that nursing was a much broader career and I liked that it was holistic. I realized that I could also obtain an advanced degree and pursue psychiatry if I still was interested. So, I moved to California to obtain my nursing degree.

What are the most rewarding aspects of your career?

I know I've touched many of my patients' lives. I am very genuine and caring in my approach to patient care. I'm also holistic and include the spiritual aspect when appropriate. I found my patients respond well to this approach and probably heal deeper than if only using the medical model. For the past year I have been working as a travel nurse and really appreciate the benefits of traveling to new places and experiencing other cultures. I also have worked as a nurse coordinator for my current travel nursing company (new company) and acted as a consultant. I've learned a lot about the business and was able to offer them my insight and knowledge as an experienced travel nurse.

Describe a typical workday in your current position.

As a travel nurse, I start a new job about every 3 months. So I'm constantly adjusting, learning, and adapting to a new environment and routine. I'm currently working on a psychiatric unit on a very busy unit. A typical day might include admitting 3 to 5 new patients, discharging a few patients, administering medications for up to 25 patients, crisis management, and facilitating groups (e.g., relaxation/guided imagery, stress management, medication education) and other nursing duties. It can be very stressful, but also rewarding.

What advice would you give to someone contemplating the same career path in nursing?

It depends whether they want to become a travel nurse or a psychiatric nurse. Travel nursing is a very exciting career. A nurse should have at least 1 year of experience in his or her specialty. Since there is very little orientation for travelers, the ability to work independently and adapt and learn quickly is highly important. In addition, they must enjoy (or don't mind) moving, and need to be flexible. Most travel nurses I know usually have an adventurous and curious spirit. Exploring new places is what makes the job fun and interesting!

How do you balance career and other aspects of your life?

I enjoy traveling and exploring different parts of the country. In my leisure time, I exercise, read, write to family, make new friends, and stay in touch with friends that I have met in my travels.

Do you have any advice for nurses who might want to purse this type of nursing career?

If you are well organized, love life, and the want the ability to move to various parts of the world, travel nursing is for you. The rewards are enormous. The main challenge for me is to figure out how to get everything I need packed into my car when I am moving to a new part of the United States, and into my luggage when I move to another country!

University Dean/President

1. **Basic description**—The university president or dean leads the faculty in fostering excellent teaching, ensuring sound scholarship, clinical expertise, and research. The university president or dean articulates the vision of the university or school through leadership in school, university, and professional activities.

2. **Educational requirements**—PhD or EdD preparation.

3. **Core competencies/skills needed:**
    *   Proven record of administrative leadership
    *   Experience in teaching nursing at a college or university level
    *   Grant writing, and/or research funding skills and experience
    *   Scholarly publications
    *   Record of service to the community/profession commensurate with the rank of associate or full professor
    *   Excellent interpersonal skills
    *   Motivation (high energy)
    *   Ability to work with others
    *   Creativity
    *   Leadership

4. **Compensation**—Varies according to place of employment and geographic location.

5. **Employment outlook**—Moderate

6. **Related Web sites and professional organizations:**
    *   Sigma Theta Tau Honor Society of Nursing: www.nursingsociety.org
    *   American Nurses Credentialing Center: www.nursingworld.org/ancc/index.htm

Women's Health Nurse

1. **Basic description**—Women's health practitioners focus on primary care for women across the life span, from adolescence to the elderly. They may be prepared for basic nursing positions or as advanced practice nurses and provide services in hospitals and a range of primary care and community based settings.

2. **Educational requirements**—RN preparation or advanced practice certification.

3. **Core competencies/skills needed:**
    -   Ability to perform well-woman assessments
    -   Instruction in self-breast exams and breast health education
    -   Knowledge of women's health
    -   Patient education
    -   Ability to provide care to women across populations, social classes, socioeconomic and age groups, and in urban, suburban, and rural settings

4. **Compensation**—Varies according to place of employment and geographic location.

5. **Employment outlook**—Moderate

6. **Related Web sites and professional organizations:**
    -   National Association for Women's Health: www.nawh.org
    -   Association of Women's Health, Obstetric and Neonatal Nurses: www.awhonn.org
    -   National Association of Nurse Practitioners in Women's Health: www.npwh.org/

Wound/Ostomy/ Continence Nurse

1. **Basic description**—An RN specializing in the care of skin, particularly involving wounds, healing, and ostomy care and appliances. Hospitals and long-term care facilities employ most of the nurses, and some work in home care.

2. **Educational requirements**—RN preparation. Certification is available through the Wound Ostomy Continence Nursing Certification Board.

3. **Core competencies/skills needed:**
   - Excellent aseptic technique
   - Excellent wound assessment skills and abilities, and wound care techniques
   - Special knowledge of wound healing and skin physiology
   - Ability to work independently and with a team
   - Excellent documentation skills
   - Knowledge of products, appliances, and wound healing
   - Responsible for dressing changes, assessment, selection of appropriate appliances, and topical wound healing, as well as pharmacological preparations
   - Skill in teaching wound care and maintenance to other staff and patients
   - Ability to maintain and promote ostomy care and teach patients to monitor their own appliances
   - Skill in patient, family, and staff education
   - Photographic documentation

4. **Compensation**—Varies according to place of employment and geographic location.

5. **Employment outlook**—Moderate
6. **Related Web sites and professional organizations:**
   - Wound, Ostomy and Continence Nurses Society: www.wocn.org
   - Wound Ostomy Continence Nursing Certification Board: www.wocncb.org/

Launching Your Career Search

Tracey Robert

DO YOU WORK TO LIVE OR LIVE TO WORK?

A simple question at first glance, but it touches at the core of defining one's self. And it forms the basis for career and life planning as we move forward into the future.

In a decade of change and upheaval, the spiritual dimension of work and career choice—the need for introspection, identifying your belief systems, and defining the role of work in your life—is and important influence in career choice. Trying to find or maintain a balanced lifestyle by integrating meaning and purpose in life with work contributes to career choice and goals. Seeking a sense of fulfillment according to shared values through your work can provide motivation and satisfaction. Planning for your career with balance in mind is important. The field of nursing can offer you the opportunity to balance your personal and professional goals in meaningful work and a quality of life. The opportunity to work at home, in the field, or in a health care facility delivering nursing care has increased the interest in the nursing profession.

Ask yourself questions like: Why am I choosing to do this type of work? Is it strictly to make money? Is it satisfying? Am I happy? What am I contributing to society? Could I be doing something else that would make me a better person? To answer the purpose in life and work question, it helps to look at some basic definitions:

Work—a series of activities including physical, intellectual, and spiritual.

Job—short-term work, can change, disappear, evolve; created by an organization to achieve its objectives and ensure orderly operations.

Career—a long-term, consistent, directed action in a chosen field; building a reputation as competent or expert; providing dignity and meaning in life through productive activity.

Spirit—the activating or essential principle influencing a person's animation; the part of you that makes meaning of life.

Purpose—having meaning, making sense of my contribution and part in the world.

Vocation—a calling.

Mission—a continuing task or responsibility that one is destined.

Can you see how the field of nursing fits into the definitions above and helps to answer the work and life question? Think about where you're headed and what's your focus? Do you work to live or live to work?

Many nurses have been drawn to the field because they want to use their skills and talents in caring for and helping others. They are able to fulfill their personal needs for contribution and purpose through the career choice of nursing.

WHY DO I NEED TO PLAN MY CAREER?

Understanding of self, the world of work, and how to connect the two happily has increased in importance. Now more than ever, work satisfaction is directly tied to both productivity and quality of life. Workers are demanding it, and work organizations can build their competitive advantage through a commitment to it.

A key element in achieving satisfaction in personal and career growth is career planning and exploration. All workers need access to the career decision-making process and need to continually assess their options if they're to thrive in an uncertain future. Career planning and development embraces three critical factors:

1. **Commitment to learning.** To meet the growing challenges of the workplace, workers need to continually upgrade skills and enhance work and life experiences through training and education. Workers, whether self-employed or working for someone else, need to dedicate themselves to "learning smart" to maintain career vitality.

Self-assessment helps workers identify strengths and weaknesses and create development plans that are future focused and productive.

The field of nursing offers multiple ways to enhance and add to the portfolio of skills required to work in the profession. A continuous opportunity for learning is what attracts many nurses to the field. The intellectual challenge and variety of tasks increases the opportunity for career satisfaction.

Curiosity for information and ideas and service provision, including professional development workshops and seminars, are an important part of the nursing profession and satisfy the need for growth and development. Career counseling and coaching, resume, interviewing, networking support and job search are available through federal, state and local agencies and the professional associations. These services provide opportunities for nurses to move among many environments in health care including international, home health care, community health just to name a few.

Self-assessment tools are available in the public and private sectors and online. A list of nationally certified career counselors is available on the web at www.nbcc.org.

2. Resilience. In a downsizing, rightsizing workforce, resilience is often required. Most workers leave their job when they perceive a lack of opportunity for development. Resilience helps them explore their options and make sound decisions.

3. Career planning. Career planning can ensure a future that has purpose and meaning versus a future of job hopping and dissatisfaction. The field of nursing has been identified as a critical employment area for the future providing multiple ways for career satisfaction and employment. Strong career planning skills can help workers identify programs and financial support for their career goals. Career planning and development is an ongoing process that targets long-range goals.

SO HOW DO I START?

Ask yourself the right questions and evaluate your answers. The right questions address concerns like what's really important to you, your priorities, what you really want and need from your work. Not the least of these concerns is finding a satisfactory balance between work and family life. These questions should include job factors such as working conditions and physical environments. The nursing profession offers a tremendous number of different working environments from the most recognizable hospital environment to international disaster sites.

Next, ask yourself what it is about your current job or experience that's failing to satisfy your needs. Determine whether it's the wrong job making you unhappy or the wrong career. Then research other jobs and career fields that you might qualify for and that might raise your level of satisfaction. Knowing why you want to enter a new career like nursing before you start is helpful. Thus armed with self-knowledge, self-awareness, and awareness of what's out there, you will be much better prepared to make sound job and career decisions.

There are basically three steps involved:

Career Self-Assessment: Know Yourself

Knowing yourself includes values, both work and personal. Identifying work and personal values can help you focus and then explore those careers that would provide fulfillment. Values of nursing include social justice, respect for the dignity of life, and professional responsibility to society. You must have interests, both work and leisure related. Nurses have expressed strong interests in helping, nurturing, and caregiving along with physical assessment knowledge and wellness. Identifying the types of patients you would like to work with and the life stages that are of interest to you are examples of the type of information needed in self-assessment.

You must have skills, including general and specific competencies and personality traits. Skills can include competencies that often transfer across different nursing practices. An example of transferring skills across nursing practice would be a nurse who initially started in the field as an emergency room nurse and then moved to a rural health clinic and is now working as a home health nurse.

COMPETENCY MEANS CAN DO

Competencies include abilities, knowledge, and attitudes that contribute to overall job performance. It pays workers to know their competencies, because:

- During the networking process this helps them identify and clarify what they have to offer and what opportunities to look for.
- Focused resumes highlighting competencies are more effective and make it easier for employers to identify a match for the organization.
- Employees who know their competencies are better able to bring their growth and development to the attention of their employers.
- Self-understanding provides a stronger basis for making career moves within or outside an organization.

Although competencies are often measured, in many cases they're confused. Not everyone agrees on what is or isn't a competency, and some say competency when they mean something else. A competency such as problem solving, for example, is usually more generic and more universal than a related skill, such as negotiation, but the latter is often called a competency.

Competencies are also confused with traits and characteristics, which include personality descriptors and distinguishing qualities that are important to a given job. For the problem-solving competency and negotiation skill, pertinent traits might include "creative" and "disciplined." And then there's style, which influences how workers use their competencies and is sometimes confused with them.

Through refinements in assessment and validation techniques, better analysis of competencies can lead to improved self-understanding and a focused job search.

IDENTIFY YOUR DECISION-MAKING STYLE

The field of nursing attracts workers who seek autonomy in their jobs and seek the opportunity to use their decision-making skills. Be able to identify how you make personal as well as work decisions.

Know your attitudes toward specific types of work environments (inside or outside) and work activity (physical or sedentary). What are your preferences about location and commuting?

Know what motivates you to work and what rewards you want from work. External rewards include compensation, benefits, and position title. Internal rewards include independence, creativity, recognition, intellectual challenge, achievement, and altruism.

Ask yourself: What are my talents, gifts, and beliefs? How can I use them in the nursing profession?

Job/Career Exploration and Industry Trends— Know the World of Work

Once you know yourself, you need to explore the world of work. What are my options? Understanding the education and training requirements for careers in nursing, typical work responsibilities, tasks required, opportunities within the field and industry, options for growth and development, viability of the field and industry, job availability, organizational culture, and environment are all important elements of this step.

Culture can be defined as the values, beliefs, and approaches shared within an organization at all levels. For employees to find the right culture fit, they must do two things: first determine and list their own workplace values, and then identify work environments that come closest to sharing them. See the government database for categories to explore and guide your search at www.doleta.gov/programs/onet

Other key sources of world of work information include

Role models and key people working in the field can help you map this out.

Informational interviewing is a key tool for a successful search.

LOOK BEFORE YOU LEAP: INFORMATION INTERVIEWS

Whether you're entering the workforce for the first time or changing jobs, industries, or careers, you need to learn about a new endeavor before you jump in: what's needed, what's expected, and what's possible. A great way to find out ahead of time which way to go is to conduct an information interview.

That means investigating a potential new position by talking with people who currently hold similar positions. Start by doing your homework, that is, conducting research to find out basic information about a particular field. Then ask around to find several possible interview subjects within that field. After you prepare a script that briefly introduces you and explains why you are calling, call them. Ask to meet with each person for a set amount of time, maybe half an hour, but be prepared to settle for a shorter phone interview if the person has limited time to give.

Opportunities for informational interviews in the field of nursing are plentiful. Professional associations can provide print and online resources for basic information and help to formulate your questions.

Since the opportunities in nursing are so plentiful, it has often been suggested that determining the age group you want to work with and the environment you would like to work in can be a starting point. The different specialty areas help direct career seekers to potential resources.

For example, a career seeker determined that he wanted to work with adolescents in an environment that would allow him to deliver direct care to patients as well as work with families. His investigation included inpatient units in a psychiatric hospital, an acute care facility dedicated to youth at risk, and a community mental health clinic working with teenagers and health promotion. All three work environments were organized differently and allowed the job candidate to explore his options and how his needs would be met. The informational interview process helps with career decisions.

The best way to kill an information interview is to ask for a job. Don't. But prepare for and conduct the interview with the same thoroughness and professionalism you would bring to a job interview. The only difference is that here you are asking the questions. Bone up before going in. Think of more questions than you need—write them down and rank them in order of importance. Key questions to ask might address the job's responsibilities, pros and cons, and the prospects for entering the field and potential for advancement. Do not hesitate to ask who else your interviewee might refer you to, and if all goes well, consider asking for a review of your resume.

As in a job interview situation, always exude confidence and professionalism. When the interview is completed, be sure to thank the interviewee for his or her time.

A great way to locate organizations that have compatible values is the direct way: ask them. Once you know which organizations you might have interest in, interview people who work there, at all levels. This is an interview in which you're conducting research to find out basic information before you make a move you might later regret. Only here you're asking which kinds of traits and behaviors thrive in a given organization and which do not. Ask for examples. And look for suppliers and customers to speak with as well as former employees. This can be especially helpful to prospective nurses to speak with other health care professionals and find out how they interact and support one another's work.

Another route to take is the Internet. Visit organizational Web sites. Or check out services that provide company reports to job applicants, such as Wet Feet Press (www.wetfeet.com) and Vault Reports (www.vaultreports.com).

Professional associations and industry conferences are rich resources for future trends in employment. Career information and online research sources can supply current information and networking sources.

NET RESULTS

Following is a review of the more useful online career resources.

JobHunt Page—(www.job-hunt.org): listings of Internet-accessible resources that could be a good starting point for a job search. They include Job Listings in Academia; Classified Advertisements; Commercial Services; Companies; University Career Resource Centers; General Job Listings; Newsgroup Searches; Other Jobs Meta-Lists; Recruiting Agencies; Reference Material; Resume Banks; Science, Engineering & Medicine.

Riley Guide—(http://www.dbm.com/jobguide): a handbook for job seekers that introduces online job information, includes beginner's information on how to conduct a job search online, catalogs recruitment Web sites and news groups by geographic location and industry and has special sections on international recruiting and resources for women and minorities.

www.careercity.com—great content on career issues and opportunity to get advice.

Job Star—(http://jobstar.org/tools/salary/): The Bay Area Library in Oakland provides links to hundreds of salary studies online, including executive summaries and sample tables.

Online Career Fairs—Participants read an employer's banner ad and can click into an employer's area for company literature, job openings and electronic applications. Here are a few:

- **Monster Board**—(www.monster.com): new series of recruitment fairs, including some geography-based or industry-based. Great for new grads!
- **CareerMosaic**—(www.careermosaic.com): allied with the Yahoo Web site to create a series of regional job fairs.

Putting It Together—Know Your Plan of Action

Goal setting and action steps will structure the planning process and make it more effective. You need to *identify goals* and strategies that will help you pursue your career direction. Generate multiple, related goals and have alternatives available. You may find multiple jobs within one profession that meet your needs and fulfill your plan. This is certainly possible in the field of nursing. Check out related occupations and resources through the Occupational Outlook Handbook at www.bls.gov/oco. The Bureau of Labor Statistics has predicted that we will need one million nurses by 2010.

Ask Yourself: What Resources Do I Need to Accomplish Each Step and the Overall Plan?

Include people, things, and data/information in your plan. Use the Internet for career information, but avoid turning this tool into a full-time job! Time spent on the Internet must be properly managed. Here are a few simple strategies to employ:

- Set aside specific times to work on your career search, and set limits on the time you spend on each session.
- Choose one topic to concentrate on, such as resumes or salaries, and stick to it throughout a session.
- Do not surf indefinitely. Go into one specific site and do a thorough search within that site. A site might hyperlink you to other sites, but that can distract and lead you down endless paths.
- There is a tendency to target employers at the start of a job search. Save that for toward the end. For a better chance of finding the right fit, first do an industry search, then career field, then job-specific listings.

Design the plan and identify barriers and possible limitations for its success. Select specific, concrete action steps that will help ensure successful completion of the plan and be true to your mission. Goal setting is hard work. Within the context of their job, people often set goals effectively. But when it comes to personal goals—this is where distractions and lack of follow-through often get in the way.

Adapting those on-the-job project management and strategic planning skills for personal development will only increase and widen opportunities for growth and development now and in the future.

Are your goals manageable and realistic? How will you keep yourself on track? How will you know you're successful? Seek out a friend or colleague that can help you brainstorm the plan and see if it fits for your purpose and makes sense. This will help you stay focused.

Making meaning is what it is all about. Map it out! Keeping a career journal will help you track your activity and keep up the momentum.

Notes From My Interview Experiences for a First Nursing Position

Nicole K. Sanders

As a new graduate interviewing for my first position as an RN, I thought I was well prepared. After all, there was an extreme nursing shortage, one that was projected to worsen. I had graduated from one of the top nursing programs and had many life experiences, both within nursing and prior to entering nursing.

I quickly discovered that there was more to learn. In talking with colleagues I also learned that new graduates often find that they do not have the skills needed to interview for their first nursing position. Here are some words of wisdom gained from my first experiences. Some of these I learned in school, and then they were reinforced in the interview process. Some I learned by the experience itself.

When you interview, wear a suit. Remember health care is a business. Always have extra copies of resumes, transcripts, and letters of reference. Bring a pen so when you are given specific information about salary and benefits you can write it down.

Be prepared to answer questions about your most acute patient, your most interesting patient, and other aspects of clinical patient care. I actually was asked very detailed questions about my clinical experiences. In my opinion, this is silly because in school we all have the same clinical rotations as students, but then, in the interview process no one asked for my opinion of the questions! It is also a good idea to remember what you learned about nursing diagnosis. Think about your strengths and weaknesses. Someone will want to know this. Be prepared for the question "Why should we hire you and what do you have to offer us?" Bite your tongue if you want to say, "You have heard that there is a nursing shortage haven't you? Why shouldn't you hire me?" In some interviews, I was asked a line of mundane questions that seemed to bore even the interviewer.

Try to get 8 hours of sleep before the interview and try to eat beforehand so that your stomach doesn't rumble! Ask questions about the mission of the institution. Remember the interview is an interaction. I believe the interviewers like it when you ask questions. Do not tell them that you did not like nursing school or that you do not particularly like taking care of sick people. Your sarcasm may not be well received. And, I have found that you have to be persistent. Sometimes it seemed as if it took a very long time for people to get back to me with a specific offer. I know that health care organizations want to make certain that the person they hire is the best "fit" for the organization. I did not realize that orientation costs are astronomical and when someone is hired and quits, it is a huge financial loss.

Plan to stay at your first job for 1 to 2 years in order to establish the rewards that one gets from feeling comfortable and competent. Be aware that most staff nursing positions require weekend and evening and night shifts, but the positive aspects of these hours are that time can be accumulated for long weekends and special activities.

I now have my first nursing position and I love it! I can see that I have chosen the career to last me a lifetime and I cannot begin to tell how rewarding it is to help those in need.

Appendix: Certification Guide

SPECIALTY CERTIFICATION BOARD	TITLE	REQUIREMENTS
ADDICTIONS NURSING CARN Certification Center for Nursing Education and Testing 601 Pavonia Avenue, Suite 201 Jersey City, NJ 07306 ($n = 963$)	CARN	Must have 3 years of experience practicing as an RN and 4,000 hours of addictions nursing practice as an RN within the past 5 years. Experience may be as a staff nurse, administrator, educator, consultant, counselor, private practitioner, or researcher. Fees: NNSA members, $175; nonmembers, $260. Valid for 4 years; may retake exam or document continuing education.

Reprinted with permission from "Your Guide to Certification," in *The American Journal of Nursing Career Guide,* January 2003, pp. 56–68. Copyright by Lippincott, Williams & Wilkins.

**CHILDBIRTH
EDUCATORS**

Lamaze International 2025 M Street, NW, Suite 800 Washington, DC 20036 www.lamaze.org ($n = 3,600$)	LCCE (formerly ACCE)	Must be a graduate of a Lamaze-accredited childbirth educator program; or currently licensed RN, CNM, RPT, MD; or awarded a baccalaureate or higher degree from a recognized institute of higher education; or be a graduate from another childbirth educator program (i.e., ICEA, Bradley, Best). You will also need documentation of 3 years of childbirth education teaching experience within the past 5 years, consisting of at least 144 instructional hours; and documentation of 30 contact hours of continuing education applicable to childbirth education within the past 3 years. Fees: Lamaze International members, $225; nonmembers, $350.

**CRITICAL CARE
NURSING**

AACN Certification Corporation 101 Columbia Aliso Vejo, CA 92656-1491		Fees: AACN members, CCRN, $220; CCNS, $325; nonmembers, CCRN, $300 (valid for 3 years), CCNS, $425 (valid for 4 years); may retake exam or document continuing education.
Adult Critical-Care Nurse ($n = 44,079$)	CCRN	Must have been actively involved in the care of critically ill adult patients. Must have a minimum of 1,750 hours within the 2 years preceding application, with 875 hours in the year previous to application. Current unrestricted RN license in the U.S.
Clinical Nurse Specialist in Acute and Critical Care; Adult, Neonatal, or Pediatric	CCNS	Must have a current unrestricted RN license in U.S.; a master's degree in nursing with evidence of CNS theory and clinical concentration in the care of the acutely or critically ill patient; and 500 hours in direct clinical practice (within the master's program or as a CNS). Recertify by exam or by completing a personal portfolio based on a self-assessment of learning needs.

Neonatal Critical-Care Nurse (*n* = 522)	CCRN	Must have been actively involved in the care of critically ill neonatal patients. Must have a minimum of 1,750 hours within the 2 years preceding application, with 875 hours in the year previous to application. Current unrestricted RN license in the U.S.
Pediatric Critical-Care Nurse (*n* = 1,307)	CCRN	Must have been actively involved in the care of critically ill pediatric patients. Must have a minimum of 1,750 hours within the 2 years preceding application, with 875 hours in the year previous to application. Current unrestricted RN license in the U.S.

DIABETES EDUCATORS

National Certification Board for Diabetes Educators 330 East Algonquin Road, Suite 4 Arlington Heights, IL 60005 www.ncbde.org (*n* = 11,785)	CDE	Must hold current unrestricted U.S. license or registration as an RN, RD, physician, pharmacist, podiatrist, PA, PT, OT, or be a health care professional with a minimum of a master's degree from an accredited U.S. college or university in: nutrition, social work, clinical psychology, exercise physiology, health education, or specified concentrations in public health. Must be currently practicing in diabetes self-management education within the U.S. or its territories. Must have completed a minimum of 2 years (24 months) of experience as a diabetes educator and a minimum of 1,000 hours of professional practice experience in diabetes self-management education within the U.S. or its territories over a period of no less than 2 years and no more than 5 years after meeting education requirements, and before applying for the certification exam. Fees: $250. Valid for 5 years; must retake the exam.

EMERGENCY NURSING

Board of Certification for Emergency Nursing 915 Lee Street Des Plaines, IL 60016 (*n* = 26,000)	CEN	Must have current unrestricted RN license. Recommended: 2 years' experience in emergency nursing practice. Valid 4 years.

FLIGHT NURSING

Board of Certification for   CFRN   Must have current unrestricted RN li-
Flight Nursing   cense. Recommended: 2 years' experience
915 Lee Street   in flight nursing practice. Valid 4 years.
Des Plaines, IL 60016

GASTROENTEROLOGY

Certifying Board of Gas-   CGN   Must have worked in gastroenterology for
troenterology Nurses   CGRN   2 years full time or its part-time equiva-
and Associates, Inc.   lent within the past 5 years or 4,000
3525 North Ellicott Mills   hours.
Drive, Suite N   Fees: SGNA members, $300; nonmem-
Ellicott City, MD 21043   bers, $350. Valid for 5 years; must retake
www.cbgna.org   the exam or recertify with 100 contact
($n = 3,000$)   hours.

**HEALTH CARE
QUALITY**

Healthcare Quality Certi-   CPHQ   Interdisciplinary for RNs, medical records
fication Board   technologists, physicians, other clinicians
PO Box 1880   and managers. Must have a minimum of
San Gabriel, CA 91778   an associate's degree. Alternate eligibility
www.cphq.org   preapplication review is available. Must
($n = 7,500$)   have practiced 2 years in health care quality, case-, utilization- and/or risk-manage-
ment activities within the last 5 years by
date of exam.
Fees: NAHQ members, $285; nonmem-
bers, $350. Recertification: 30 CE hours
every 2 years. Valid for 2 years.

HIV/AIDS NURSING

HIV/AIDS Nursing Certi-   ACRN   Must hold current license as RN in the
fication Board   U.S., or international equivalent, and have
c/o Professional Testing   2 years of experience in clinical practice,
Corporation   education, management, or research in
1350 Broadway   HIV/AIDS nursing. Valid for 4 years. Re-
New York, NY 10018   certification: Retake the exam or acquire
40 CEUs.
Fees: ANAC members, $200; nonmem-
bers, $350.

HOLISTIC NURSING

American Holistic Nurses' Certification Corp.
5102 Ganymede Drive
Austin, TX 78727
helenerickson@mail.utexas.edu

HNC

Must have current unrestricted license as an RN. Must have minimum of a baccalaureate. Minimum of 1 year full-time practice as a holistic nurse or part-time for a minimum of 2,000 hours within last 5 years. Minimum of 48 contact hours of continuing education in areas of holistic nursing. Must meet criteria for qualitative assessment and pass the national exam. Call toll free, (877) 284-0998, for information.

Fees: $25 application; $150 qualitative assessment; $210 quantitative test. Valid for 5 years; recertification with 100 CE hours of which 20 must be in holistic nursing. The remaining 80 hours can be related to holistic modalities, methods of practice, and studies that facilitate self-care, growth, and transformation within a holistic context.

HOSPICE AND PALLIATIVE NURSING

National Board for Certification of Hospice and Palliative Nurses
Penn Center West One, Suite 229
Pittsburgh, PA 15276
nbchpn@hpna.org
(*n* = 5,000)

CHPN

Must be currently licensed as an RN in the U.S. or the equivalent in Canada; at least 2 years of experience in hospice and palliative nursing practice recommended. Fees: HPNA members, $230; nonmembers, $330; renewal: members, $195; nonmembers, $295.

INFECTION CONTROL

Certification Board of Infection Control and Epidemiology, Inc.
1275 K Street, NW, Suite 1000
Washington, DC 20005-4006
info@cbic.org
www.cbic.org
(*n* = 4,100)

CIC

Have a current license or registration as an RN, medical technologist, or physician. Must have a minimum of a baccalaureate in a health care–related field. There is a waiver process for candidates who do not meet the education requirements. Must have practiced infection control for a minimum of 2 years.

Fees: $295; recertification, $245. Valid for 5 years; may retake the exam or the Self-Assessment Recertification Examination (SARE).

INFUSION NURSING

Infusion Nurses Certification Corporation
220 Norwood Park South
Norwood, MA 02062
www.insl.org
(*n* = 3,600)

CRNI

Candidate must have a minimum of 1,600 hours of experience as an RN in infusion therapy within the last 2 years prior to date of application, a current RN license in the U.S. or Canada, and must complete the CRNI examination registration form. Fees: INS members, $250; nonmembers, $400. Recertification every 3 years by exam or by continuing education.

LACTATION CONSULTANT

International Board of Lactation Consultant Examiners
7309 Arlington Boulevard, Suite 300
Falls Church, VA 22042-3215
(*n* = 8,000)

IBCLC

Must have 30 hours of education specific to breastfeeding within 3 years prior to taking the exam. Those with a baccalaureate or higher degree must have 2,500 BC practice hours; those with 60 academic credits (associate degree or RN diploma) must have 4,000 hours of practice. Alternate pathways are available.
Fees: $395. Valid for 5 years; recertification by exam or by continuing education; every 10 years by exam only.

LEGAL NURSE CONSULTING

American Legal Nurse Consultant Certification Board*
4700 West Lake Avenue
Glenview, IL 60025-1485
info@aalnc.org
www.aalnc.org
(*n* = 346)

LNCC

Must possess a full and unrestricted license as an RN in the U.S. or its territories; have a bachelor's degree or the equivalent of 5 years' experience as a legal nurse consultant; have practiced 2 years as an RN; have evidence of 2,000 hours of legal nurse consulting experience within the 3 years prior to the application.
Fees: AALNC members, $275; nonmembers, $375. Valid for 5 years; may retake the exam or CE credits.

NEPHROLOGY NURSING

Board of Nephrology

CHN

Must have current U.S. license; technolo-

---

*Has met the standards of the American Board of Nursing Specialties, a national peer review program.

Examiners	CPDN	gists must have high school diploma or equivalent; both must have 1 year experience in caring for patients with end-stage renal disease.
Nursing and Technology (BONENT) PO Box 15945-282 Lenexa, KS 66285	CHT	

Fees: Exam, $195, annual fee, $50. Recertification every 4 years, must submit documentation of 45 CEUs (30 nephrology-related) every 4 years or retake exam.

Nephrology Nursing Certification Commission
East Holly Avenue, PO Box 56
Pitman, NJ 08071-0056   **CNN**

Must possess a BSN; hold full, unrestricted RN license in U.S. or its territories. Three years prior to application must have minimum 2 years' nephrology nursing experience as RN in general staff, administrative, teaching, or research (at least 50% of employment hours in nephrology nursing); and complete 30 CEUs for fundamental nephrology nursing.
Fees: ANNA members, $175; nonmembers, $225. Valid for 3 years. May recertify by accruing 60 CE contact hours during that period, or retake the test.

CDN

Must hold current, full, unrestricted RN license in U.S. or its territories; complete a minimum of 2,000 hours as an RN in nephrology nursing during the last 2 years; complete 15 hours of approved CE in nephrology nursing within 2 years prior to submission of application.
Fees: ANNA members, $175; nonmembers, $225 (includes $50 nonrefundable application processing fee). Valid 3 years. Recertify with exam or CE credits.

CCHT

Must possess a minimum of a high school diploma or GED; have successfully completed a training program for hemodialysis patient care technicians that included classroom instruction and supervised clinical experience; obtain the signature of a preceptor/supervisor to verify training and clinical experience (minimum 6 months or 1,000 hours clinical experience recommended prior to taking exam); be in compliance with state regulations.
Fees: exam, $125 (includes $25 nonrefundable application processing fee).
Valid 2 years. Recertify with exam or CE credits.

**NEUROSCIENCE
NURSING**
American Board of   CNRN   Must have 2 years of experience in neuro-
Neuroscience   science nursing. Must be engaged in clini-
Nursing   cal practice or as a consultant, researcher,
4700 W Lake Avenue   administrator, or educator in neurosci-
Glenview, IL 60025   ence nursing.
(*n* = 1,500)   Fees: AANN members, $215; nonmem-
                                                bers, $300. Valid for 5 years; may recer-
                                                tify through CE units or retake the exam.

**NURSE
ADMINISTRATION—
LONG-TERM CARE**
NADONA/LTC Certifica-   CDONA/   Must be a director of nursing administra-
tion Registrar   LTC   tion in a long-term care setting for at
10999 Reed Hartman   least 12 months in the previous 5 years.
Highway, Suite 233   Former DONs and assistant DONs are eli-
Cincinnati, OH 45242-   gible to take the exam.
8301   Fees: NADONA/LTC members, $125; non-
(*n* = 4,000)   members, $200. Valid for 5 years; recer-
                                                tify with a $60 fee and validation of 75
                                                hours of continuing education every 5
                                                years.

NURSE ANESTHETIST
Council on Certification   CRNA   Must be a graduate of a nurse anesthesia
of Nurse Anesthetists*   educational program accredited by the
222 South Prospect Av-   Council on Accreditation of Nurse Anes-
enue   thesia Educational Programs and maintain
Park Ridge, IL 60068-   current unrestricted RN license in the
5790   U.S. and its territories. Must certify that
scaulk@aana.com   RN license is not currently and has not
(*n* = 26,000)   been subject to investigation or legal ac-
                                                tion, and that individual has no mental,
                                                physical, or other problems that could in-
                                                terfere with the practice of anesthesia.
                                                Fees: $550. Recertify every 2 years; docu-
                                                ment 40 hours of approved continuing ed-
                                                ucation; document substantial
                                                engagement in nurse anesthesia practice;
                                                maintain current unrestricted RN licen-
                                                sure; certify that RN license is not cur-
                                                rently and has not been subject to
                                                investigation or legal action.

---

*Has met the standards of the American Board of Nursing Specialties, a national peer review pro-
gram.

**NURSE MIDWIFERY
AND MIDWIFERY**

ACNM Certification   CNM   Satisfactory completion of an accredited
Council, Inc.   CM   midwifery program. Exam must be taken
8401 Corporate Drive,   within 12 months of completing the pro-
Suite 630   gram. Recertify every 8 years by (option
Landover, MD 20785   1) completing 3 ACC certificate mainte-
(n = 8,400)   nance modules (antepartum, intrapartum/
newborn and postpartum/gynecology),
and accruing 2 CEUs of ACNM or AC-
CME Category 1 approved activities; or
(option 2) passing exam and accruing 2
CEUs of ACNM or ACCME Category 1
approved activities.
Fees: $425 for initial exam; $55 per year
for certificate maintenance.

**NUTRITION SUPPORT
NURSING**

National Board of Nutri-   CNSN   Must be a currently licensed RN in the
tion Support Certifica-   U.S. or the equivalent in other countries.
tion   Candidates should have at least 2 years'
American Society for Par-   experience in specialized nutrition sup-
enteral and Enteral Nutri-   port.
tion   Fees: ASPEN members, $225; nonmem-
8630 Fenton Street,   bers, $275. Valid for 5 years. Recertify by
Suite 412   retaking and passing exam.
Silver Spring, MD
20910-3805
www.nutritioncare.org
(n = 161)

**OCCUPATIONAL
HEALTH NURSING**

American Board for Oc-   COHN   Must prove 50 course contact hours in occupational Health   COHN-S   cupational health, or in courses related to
Nurses, Inc.*   occupational health, taken within the pre-
201 East Ogden, Suite   ceding 5 years; have 2 years (4,000
114   hours) of experience in occupational
Hinsdale, IL 60521-3652   health nursing; have valid nursing license;
www.abohn.org   be employed minimum of 8 hours a week
(n = 6,700)   in occupational health nursing. Individual
consideration is given to occupational
health nurses who meet the experience criteria but are currently enrolled full time

*Has met the standards of the American Board of Nursing Specialties, a national peer review pro-
gram.

in a graduate program of study in occupational health nursing or in a related field.
For COHN-S, a baccalaureate degree in
nursing is required.
Fees: application, $50; exam, $275; recertification, $225. Valid for 5 years; recertify
with 75 CE hours in occupational health
and 4,000 hours of work experience or
100 CE hours and 3,000 hours of work
experience.

| Occupational Health Nurse Case Manager | COHN/CM COHN-S/CM | Must have current COHN or COHN-S, current nursing license, and 10 CE hours incase management in past 5 years. Fees: application, $35; exam, $150; recertification, $100. Valid for 5 years; recertify with 10 CE hours in occupational health, case management, and continued base certification. |

ONCOLOGY NURSING

| Oncology Nursing Certification Corporation* 501 Holiday Drive Pittsburgh, PA 15220-2749 www.oncc.org (n = 17,855) | OCN | Must have minimum of 12 months of experience as an RN within the last 3 years, 1,000 hours of oncology nursing practice within the last 30 months, and current RN license. Fees: ONS members, $220; nonmembers, $320. Valid for 4 years; may renew every other cycle by ONC-PRO; must take test at least every 8 years. Recertification: ONS members, $170; nonmembers, $270. |
| (n = 1,007) | AOCN | Must have minimum of 30 months of experience as an RN within the 5 years prior to application, 2,000 hours of oncology nursing practice within the past 5 years, current license, and master's degree or higher in nursing. Fees: ONS members, $250; nonmembers, $350. Valid for 4 years; may renew every other cycle by ONC-PRO; must take test at least every 8 years. Recertification: ONS members, $200; nonmembers, $300. |

*Has met the standards of the American Board of Nursing Specialties, a national peer review program.

OPHTHALMIC NURSING

National Certifying Board for Ophthalmic Registered Nurses PO Box 193030 San Francisco, CA 94119 www.asom.org (*n* = 350)	CRNO	Must have at least 2 years of full-time (4,000 hours) experience in ophthalmic nursing practice. Fees: ASORN members, $275; nonmembers, $350. Valid for 5 years; must retake exam document 75 CE hours.

ORTHOPAEDIC NURSING

Orthopaedic Nurses Certification Board* East Holly Avenue, PO Box 56 Pitman, NJ 08071 (*n* = 3,300)	ONC	Must have 2 years of experience practicing as an RN holding a current and unrestricted license, and 1,000 hours of work experience in orthopaedic nursing practice within past 3 years. Fees: NAON members, $205; nonmembers, $285. Valid for 5 years; may retake the exam or document 100 continuing education hours.

PAIN MANAGEMENT

American Academy of Pain Management 13947 Mono Way #A Sonora, CA 95370	FAAPM	Interdisciplinary with 3 levels of certification. Nurses who are doctorally prepared earn diplomate; nurses with a master's degree earn a fellow. Both must have 2 years of experience working with patients who have pain. Baccalaureate-prepared nurses earn clinical associate status and must have 5 years of relevant experience in pain management. All must submit 3 letters of professional reference, official academic transcripts, curriculum vitae, license, and application. Must also pass the certification exam. Fees: $250 (general membership, $150; application, $100); exam, $175; annual renewal, $150. Valid for 4 years; recertify by documenting 100 contact hours of continuing education.

---

*Has met the standards of the American Board of Nursing Specialties, a national peer review program.

PEDIATRIC NURSING

National Certification   CPN
Board of Pediatric Nurse
Practitioners & Nurses
800 South Frederick Ave-
nue, Suite 104
Gaithersburg, MD
20877-41150
info@pnpcert.org
www.pnpcert.org
($n = 4,300$)

Must provide documentation of current RN licensure in U.S. and completion of basic RN education (diploma, associate, baccalaureate, or master's degree). Must document 2 years of full-time or equivalent experience (total 3,600 hours minimum) as an RN in a pediatric nursing specialty in a U.S. facility within the past 4 years, including direct patient care, teaching, administration, clinical research, or consultation in pediatric nursing.
Fees: $260. Valid for 5 years; renewed annually by documentation of 10 CEUs or 1 academic credit in pediatric nursing, or re-examination within 5 years of certification. All exams are computer based, given year round through Prometric/Sylvan Technology Testing Centers.

($n = 7,800$)   CPNP

Must be a graduate of a PNP master's, post-master's, or doctorate program recognized by NCBPNP/N and submit documentation including transcripts showing degrees conferred. Must pass exam within 24 months after completing program. An alternative pathway and certification by endorsement are also offered.
Fees: $375. Annual certification maintenance through self-assessment exercise, 10 CEUs/year, and/or documentation of clinical PNP practice. All exams are computer based, given year round through Prometric/Sylvan Technology Testing Centers.

PEDIATRIC
ONCOLOGY

Oncology Nursing Certi-   CPON
fication Corporation
501 Holiday Drive
Pittsburgh, PA.15220-
2749
www.oncc.org
($n = 650$)

Must have minimum of 12 months' experience as RN, 1,000 hours pediatric oncology nursing practice within past 30 months, and current RN license.
Fees: ONS or APON members, $250; nonmembers, $350. Valid for 4 years. Recertification: members, $200; nonmembers, $300. After passing ONCC-administered CPON exam, may renew every other year by ONC-PRO. Must retake test every 8 years.

PERIANESTHESIA NURSING

The American Board of Perianesthesia Nursing Certification, Inc.
475 Riverside Drive, 7th Floor
New York, NY 10115-0089
abpanc@proexam.org
www.cpancapa.org
Certified Post Anesthesia Nurse
(n = 5,439 CPNA; n = 1,506 CAPA)

CPAN
CAPA

Candidates applying for CPAN or CAPA certification must hold a current unrestricted RN license and have a minimum of 1,800 hours of direct perianesthesia practice experience as an RN during the past 2 consecutive years. Nurses working as direct caregiver, manager, teacher, or researcher in perianesthesia are eligible for certification.
Candidates may contact ABPANC's national office to inquire which certification exam would be appropriate for them.
Fees: ASPAN member, $235; nonmember, $335; recertification: member, $150; nonmember, $280. Certification valid for 3 years; recertification by examination or continuing learning program.

PERIOPERATIVE NURSING

Certification Board of Perioperative Nursing
2170 South Parker Road, Suite 295
Denver, CO 80231-5710
(n = 28,700)

CNOR

Must have a minimum of 2 full years and 2,400 hours of operating room practice as an RN; been employed within the previous 2 years, either full time or part time as an RN in an administrative, teaching, research, or general staff capacity in perioperative nursing.
Fees: AORN members, $250; nonmembers, $350. Valid for 5 years; may retake the exam or document 125 contact hours of approved CE.

RN First Assistant
(n =1,650)

CRNFA

Must be certified as a CNOR; must document 2,000 hours of practice in the RN first assistant role, with at least 500 hours in the past 2 years; must have attended a formal RNFA program; must be BSN prepared.
Fees: AORN members, $375; nonmembers, $500. Valid for 5 years; may retest or submit continuing education to recertify.

**PLASTIC AND
RECONSTRUCTIVE
SURGICAL NURSING**

Plastic Surgical Nursing Certification Board East Holly Avenue, PO Box 56 Pitman, NJ 08071 ($n = 425$)	CPSN	Must have a minimum of 2 years of experience in plastic surgical nursing as an RN in a general staff, administrative, teaching, or research capacity within 5 years prior to application, and have spent at least 50% of practice hours in plastic surgical nursing during 2 of the preceding 5 years. Fees: ASPRSN members, $195; nonmembers, $295. Recertification: members, $135; nonmembers, $185. Valid for 3 years; may retake the exam or obtain 45 contact hours of continuing education with a minimum of 30 in plastic surgical nursing.

**REHABILITATION
NURSING**

Rehabilitation Nursing Certification Board* 4700 West Lake Avenue Glenview, IL 60025-1485 www.rehabnurse.org ($n = 12,500$)	CRRN	Must have current, unrestricted RN license; minimum of 2 years of practice as an RN in rehabilitation nursing in the last 5 years. Fees: ARN members, $195; nonmembers, $285. Valid for 5 years; retake the exam or recertify by 60 points of credit with a combination of continuing education, presentations, professional publications, formal course work, and/or submitting test items.
	CRRN-A	Must be CRRN with an unrestricted nursing license and master's degree in nursing or doctorate in nursing. Fees: ARN members, $240; nonmembers, $320. Valid for 5 years.

---

*Has met the standards of the American Board of Nursing Specialties, a national peer review program.

SCHOOL NURSING

National Board of Certifi- NCSN
cation of School Nurses,
Inc.
PO Box 1300
Scarborough, ME 04070-
1300
nasn@nasn.org
(*n* = 1,500)

Must be currently licensed as an RN with
a 4-year degree. Three years of experience
as a school nurse recommended.
Fees: NASN members, $175; nonmem-
bers, $250.

UROLOGY NURSING

Certification Board for CURN
Urologic Nurses and As- CUA
sociates CUNP
East Holly Avenue, PO CUCNS
Box 56 CUPA
Pitman, NJ 08071-0056
(*n* = 519)

RN, LPN, LVN, PA: current licensure and
1 year experience in urology nursing practice. Other associates: 3 years' in-service
training under supervision of a practicing
urologist. Advanced practice: same as RN,
but with current recognition by state
board of nursing as nurse practitioner
and/or clinical nurse specialist, and an
earned master's degree in nursing.
Fees: SUNA members, $195; nonmem-
bers, $255; advanced practice SUNA mem-
bers, $225; nonmembers, $285. Valid for
3 years; may either retest or provide proof
of 50 contact hours.

WOMEN'S HEALTH NURSING

National Certification
Corporation for the Ob-
stetric, Gynecologic and
Neonatal Nursing Spe-
cialties
PO Box 11082
Chicago, IL 60611-0082
www.nccnet.org

For all categories, must have experience/
employment in direct patient care, education, administration, and/or research.
Written exam given 4 times a year; Valid
for 3 years. Certification Maintenance Program requires 45 contact hours of approved CE or re-examination for RNC,
and 15 hours approved CE or re-exam for
subspecialty.

Breastfeeding
(*n* = 826)

Must pass subspecialty exam; be licensed
RN in the U.S. or Canada; be employed.
Pathway 1: Must be certified by NCC,
ACNM, or ANCC. Pathway 2: Must have
24 months of practice in the specialty.
Fees: NCC RNCs, $100; non-NCC RNCs,
$135.

Electronic Fetal Monitoring (n = 826)		Must pass subspecialty exam; be licensed RN, MD, or physician's assistant in the U.S. or Canada. Fees: NCC RNCs, $100; non-NCC RNCs, $135.
Inpatient Obstetric Nurse (n = 35,147)	RNC	For the following specialties: must be a licensed RN in the U.S. or Canada and have 24 months of experience in the specialty, including a minimum of 2,000 hours as an RN. Employment within the last 24 months is required. Fee: $250.
Low Risk Neonatal Nurse (n = 5,336)	RNC	
Maternal Newborn Nurse (n = 4,275)	RNC	
Neonatal Intensive Care Nurse (n = 13,979)	RNC	
Neonatal Nurse Practitioner (n = 4,276)	RNC	Must be a licensed RN in the U.S. or Canada; graduate from a master's or post-master's degree neonatal nurse practitioner program at least 1 academic year in length and acceptable to NCC; have 200 didactic hours and 600 clinical hours.
Primary Care Nurse Practitioner—Obstetrics (n = 9)		Must be a licensed RN in the U.S. or Canada; be certified by ANCC, AANP, or NCBPNP. Current employment required. Fee: $135.
Primary Care Nurse Practitioner—Gynecology/ Reproductive Health Care (n = 42)		Must be a licensed RN in the U.S. or Canada; be certified by ANCC, AANP, or NCBPNP. Current employment required. Fee: $135.
Women's Health Care Nurse Practitioner (n = 13,016)	RNC	Must be a licensed RN in the U.S. or Canada; graduate from a women's health care nurse practitioner program that is at least 1 academic year in length and is acceptable to NCC; have 200 didactic hours and 600 clinical hours. Effective January 1, 2007, a graduate degree will be required.

**AMERICAN NURSES
CREDENTIALING
CENTER**
600 Maryland Avenue,
SW, Suite 100 West
Washington, DC 20024-
2571

*Clinical specialist and nurse practitioner
candidates* must hold an active RN license
in the U.S. or its territories; hold a master's or higher degree in nursing (see ex-
ceptions for Psychiatric and Mental
Health Nursing and Community Health
Nursing). Must have been prepared in the
area of practice through a master's program or a formal postgraduate master's
program in nursing that includes both didactic and clinical components and a minimum of 500 hours of supervised clinical
practice in the specialty area and is offered by a school of nursing that grants
graduate-level academic credit for all of
the course work.

Specialty nursing certification candidates
must hold an active RN license in the
U.S. or its territories; have practiced the
equivalent of 2 years full-time as an RN
in the U.S. or its territories; hold a baccalaureate or higher degree in nursing; have
a minimum of 2,000 hours of clinical
practice within the last 3 years, unless
specified in criteria specific to the specialty area. Must have had 30 contact
hours within the last 3 years. Faculty may
use up to 500 hours of teaching or clinical supervision in the specialty area of
practice toward the practice requirement.
Students may use up to 500 hours of time
spent in an academic program of nursing
study toward their clinical practice requirement.

Modular certification candidates must meet
one of the following sets of basic eligibility requirements. CORE certified nurses
must hold an active RN license in the
U.S. or its territories; show proof of a current, nationally recognized, core nursing
specialty certification, and have functioned within the specialty scope of practice for a minimum of 2,000 hours within

the last 2 years. Non-core certified nurses must hold an active RN license in the U.S. or its territories and have functioned as an RN for 4,000 hours, with at least 2,000 of them within the specialty scope of practice, within the last 2 years. Fees: (written exam) ANA members, $180; discount (members of other associations), $250; nonmembers, $320; (computer-based exam) members, $230; discount, $300; nonmembers, $370.

Acute Care Nurse Practitioner CS
(*n* = 879)

Must meet basic eligibility requirements.

Adult Nurse Practitioner* CS
(*n* = 9,571)

Must hold a master's or higher degree in nursing. Must have been prepared as an adult nurse practitioner (ANP) in either an ANP master's degree in nursing program or a family nurse practitioner master's degree in nursing program; or a formal postgraduate ANP or family nurse practitioner track or program within a school of nursing granting graduate-level academic credit.

Cardiac and Vascular Nurse* C
(*n* = 348)

Must hold a baccalaureate or higher degree in nursing. Must have practiced as a licensed RN for a minimum of 2 years; provide evidence of successful completion of American Heart Association ACLS program; currently practice in a cardiac rehabilitation setting an average of 8 hours per week; have a minimum of 2,000 hours of hospital experience either in critical care or acute coronary care; have 30 contact hours of continuing education applicable to cardiac rehabilitation within the past 3 years.

---

*Has met the standards of the American Board of Nursing Specialties, a national peer review program.

Case Management (Exam 30) (Modular Certification)	Cm	Must have a core nursing specialty certification. Must hold a baccalaureate or higher degree in nursing; have functioned within the scope of an RN case manager a minimum of 2,000 hours within the past 2 years.
Case Management (Exam 31) (Modular Certification)	Cm	For candidates who do not hold a core nursing specialty certification: must hold a baccalaureate or higher degree in nursing; have functioned as an RN for 4,000 hours, with at least 2,000 of those hours as a nurse case manager within the past 2 years.
Clinical Specialist in Adult Psychiatric Mental Health Nursing* ($n = 6,700$) Clinical Specialist in Child and Adolescent Psychiatric and Mental Health Nursing* ($n = 883$)	CS	Candidates who do not have a master's or higher degree in psychiatric and mental health nursing must hold a master's or higher degree in nursing, with a minimum of 18 graduate or postgraduate academic credits in PMH theory. A minimum of 9 of these credits must contain didactic and clinical experiences specific to PMH nursing theory. A maximum of 9 of the credits may be in courses containing didactic and clinical experiences specific to PMH theory. Must have supervised clinical training at the graduate or postgraduate level in 2 psychotherapeutic treatment modalities.
Clinical Specialist in Community Health Nursing* ($n = 412$)	CS	In addition to the basic requirements, may have either a master's or higher degree in community health nursing or a baccalaureate degree in nursing and a master's or higher degree in public health with a specialization in community/public health nursing. The specialization must be verified by a letter from the institution where the degree was obtained or by a statement on the official transcript.
Clinical Specialist in Gerontological Nursing* ($n = 854$)	CS	Must hold a master's or higher degree in gerontological nursing; or with a specialization in gerontological nursing. Must have practiced 12 months following com-

*Has met the standards of the American Board of Nursing Specialties, a national peer review program.

pletion of the master's degree. If a clinical specialist, must have provided 800 hours (post-master's) of direct patient care or clinical management in gerontological nursing in the past 24 months. If a consultant, researcher, educator, or administrator, must have provided 400 hours (post-master's) of direct patient care or clinical management in gerontological nursing in the past 24 months.

Clinical Specialist in Home Health Nursing (*n* = 61)	CS	Must hold a master's or higher degree in nursing and within the past 24 months have practiced as a licensed RN in Home Health Nursing a minimum of 1,000 hours (post-master's). If graduated from a CS in Home Health Nursing program, 50% of the clinical practice within the graduate program may be applied toward the 1,000-hour practice requirement. Must currently provide at least 8 hours per week of direct patient care or clinical management in home health nursing.
Clinical Specialist in Medical-Surgical Nursing* (*n* = 2,182)	CS	Must hold a master's degree in nursing with evidence of medical-surgical concentration; be currently providing direct patient care in medical-surgical nursing an average of 4 hours or more weekly; have practiced 12 months following completion of the master's degree; have provided 800 hours of direct patient care within the past 24 months. If employed as a consultant, researcher, administrator, or educator, must have provided direct patient care in medical-surgical nursing 400 hours (post-master's) within the past 24 months.

*Has met the standards of the American Board of Nursing Specialties, a national peer review program.

College Health Nurse* (*n* = 1,003)	C	Must hold a baccalaureate or higher degree in nursing; have a minimum of 1,500 hours of practice as a licensed RN in college health nursing; and currently practice college health nursing an average of 8 hours per week (minimum of 288 hours per year). Must have 30 contact hours of continuing education in specialty in past 3 years.
Community Health Nurse* (*n* = 1,867)	C	Must hold a baccalaureate or higher degree in nursing; have practiced as a licensed RN in community health nursing a minimum of 1,500 hours; have 30 contact hours of continuing education in the specialty in the past 3 years.
Family Nurse Practitioner* (*n* = 16,350)	CS	Must hold a master's or higher degree in nursing; have been prepared as a family nurse practitioner (FNP) in either an FNP master's degree in nursing program, or a formal postgraduate FNP track or program within a school of nursing granting graduate-level academic credit.
General Nursing Practice (*n* = 2,057)	CS	Must have a minimum of 4,000 hours of practice as an RN in general nursing practice. Must have practiced 2,000 hours within the last 3 years.
Gerontological Nurse* (*n* = 16,566)	C	Must hold a baccalaureate or higher degree in nursing. Must have a minimum of 4,000 hours of practice as an RN in gerontological nursing, 2,000 of which must have been within the past 2 years. (Time spent in a formal program of advanced nursing study may count toward 300 hours.) Must have had 30 contact hours of continuing education applicable to gerontology/gerontological nursing within the past 2 years. Practice requirements can be met if candidates have engaged in direct patient care or clinical management, supervision, education, or direction of others to achieve patient goals.

---

*Has met the standards of the American Board of Nursing Specialties, a national peer review program.

Gerontological Nurse Practitioner* (n = 2,813)	CS	Must hold a master's degree in nursing. Must have been prepared as a nurse practitioner in either a gerontological nurse practitioner (GNP) master's degree in nursing program or a formal postgraduate GNP track or program within a school of nursing granting graduate-level academic credit.
Home Health Nurse* (n = 1,422)	C	Must hold a baccalaureate or higher degree in nursing; have practiced as a licensed RN in home health nursing for a minimum of 1,500 hours; currently practice home health nursing a minimum of 8 hours per week; have 20 contact hours of continuing education in specialty within the past 2 years.
Informatics Nurse (n = 190)	C	Must hold a baccalaureate or higher degree in nursing and an active RN license in the U.S. or its territories; have practiced as a licensed RN for a minimum of 2 years; have practiced at least 2,000 hours in the field of informatics nursing within the past 5 years, or have completed at least 12 semester hours of academic credits in informatics in a graduate program in informatics nursing within the past 5 years, and have 20 contact hours of continuing education in specialty in the past 2 years.
Medical-Surgical Nurse* (n = 33,818)	C	Must hold a baccalaureate or higher degree in nursing. Must have practiced a minimum of 4,000 hours as an RN in medical-surgical nursing, with 2,000 hours within the past 2 years, and currently practice medical-surgical nursing an average of 8 hours per week. Requirements may be met if engaged in direct patient care or clinical management, supervision, education, or direction of others to achieve patient goals. Also must have 30 contact hours of continuing education in specialty within the past 3 years.

---

*Has met the standards of the American Board of Nursing Specialties, a national peer review program.

Nursing Administration* (n = 5,154)	CNA	Must hold an active RN license in the U.S. or its territories and hold a baccalaureate or higher degree in nursing. Must have held an administrative position at nurse manager or nurse executive level for at least the equivalent of 24 months' full-time practice within the past 5 years.
Nursing Administration, Advanced* (n = 2,091)	CNAA	Must hold an active RN license in the U.S. or its territories and a master's or higher degree. For nurses first licensed in 1990 and after, if the master's degree is not in nursing, a baccalaureate in nursing will be required. Also must have held an administrative position at the nurse executive level for at least 24 months, full-time service within the past 5 years. Must have 30 contact hours of continuing education in specialty in the past 2 years, or hold a master's degree in nursing administration. A combination of CE and academic credit, as well as presenter/lecturer credit is acceptable.
Nursing Continuing Education/Staff Development* (n = 1,843)	C	Must hold a baccalaureate or higher degree in nursing; have practiced as an RN in nursing continuing education and/or staff development for a minimum of 4,000 hours during the past 5 years; currently practice as a licensed RN in nursing continuing education and/or staff development an average of 20 hours or more per week. Must have 20 contact hours of continuing education in specialty in the past 2 years.
Pediatric Nurse* (n = 3,964)	C	Must hold a baccalaureate or higher degree in nursing. Must have at least 2,100 hours as an RN in pediatric nursing. (Time spent in a formal program of advanced nursing study may count for 300 hours.) This requirement can be met if engaged in direct patient care or clinical management, supervision, education, or

---

*Has met the standards of the American Board of Nursing Specialties, a national peer review program.

the direction of others to achieve patient goals. Also must have 30 contact hours of continuing education applicable to pediatric nursing within the past 3 years.

Pediatric Nurse Prac-   CS
titioner*
(*n* = 2,752)

In addition to meeting the basic eligibility requirements, must have graduated from a program that provides course work that addresses children's unique physiologic, psychologic, and developmental needs from birth through age 21. If graduated 3 or more years ago, must have worked 2,000 hours in a pediatric clinical position in the immediate 3 years prior to applying for exam. Submit verification of current practice with application.

Perinatal Nurse*   C
(*n* = 990)

Must hold a baccalaureate or higher degree in nursing. Must have practiced 2,100 hours as an RN in perinatal nursing in the past 3 years. (Time spent in a formal program of advanced nursing study may count for 300 hours.) This requirement can be met in direct patient care or clinical management, supervision, education, or direction of others to achieve patient goals. Also must have had 30 contact hours of continuing education in specialty within the past 3 years.

Psychiatric and Mental   C
Health Nurse*
(*n* = 22,124)

Must have current access to clinical consultation/supervision. Must provide a statement or endorsement of clinical consultation/supervision from a nurse colleague.

School Nurse   C
(*n* = 142)

Must hold a baccalaureate or higher degree in nursing. Must have completed a practice requirement in school nursing that can be met by completion of a 200-hour supervised college-sponsored internship or practicum in school nursing, or completion of 1,500 hours in school nursing practice, supervision, education, or direction of other persons engaged in

---

*Has met the standards of the American Board of Nursing Specialties, a national peer review program.

		school nursing within the past 3 years, or a combination of practicum hours and school nursing experience.
School Nurse Practitioner* (*n* = 236)	CS	Must hold a master's or higher degree in nursing. Must have been prepared as a school nurse practitioner (SNP) in either an SNP graduate nursing degree program or a formal postgraduate SNP track or program within a school of nursing granting graduate-level academic credit. Certified school nurse practitioners can recertify by continuing education only. The recertification exam option is no longer offered.

---

*Has met the standards of the American Board of Nursing Specialties, a national peer review program.

Glossary of Acronyms

ACLS Advanced Cardiac Life Support
AD Associate Degree
AHNCC The American Holistic Nurses' Certification Corporation
APRN Advanced Practice Registered Nurse
BCLS Basic Cardiac Life Support
BSN Bachelors of Science in Nursing
CCRN Critical Care Registered Nurse
CPT Current Procedural Terminology
DRG Diagnostic Related Group
ECG Electrocardiogram
ED Emergency Department
EMT Emergency Medical Technician
ER Emergency Room
FNP Family Nurse Practitioner
GNP Geriatric Nurse Practitioner
IBCLC International Board Certified Lactation Consultant
IBLCE International Board of Lactation Consultant Examiners
LNC Legal Nurse Consultant
LPN Licensed Practical Nurse
MI Myocardial Infarction
MSN Masters of Science in Nursing
MPH Masters in Public Health
OSHA Occupational Safety & Health Administration
PNP Pediatric Nurse Practitioner
RHIA Registered Health Information Technition
RN Registered Nurse
RRA Record Review Auditor
SANE Sexual Assault Nurse Examiner
SNF Skilled Nursing Facilities
TB Tuberculosis

Springer Publishing Company

From the Springer Series: Teaching of Nursing...

A Nuts-and-Bolts Approach to Teaching Nursing, *2nd Edition*

Victoria Schoolcraft, MSN, RN, PhD
with Jeanne Novotny, PhD, RN

"The book is 'must' reading for new faculty...It is also an excellent review for seasoned faculty who might need a refresher course on teaching nursing." —**Journal of Professional Nursing**

Here is the revised and updated edition of this down-to-earth survival manual for those who are teaching for a brief time, for those who are new to teaching, and for those who need a quick refresher course.

Brimming with practical pointers and dozens of timesaving tables and checklists, this precise volume delineates strategies you will need to make clinical assignments, select the right textbook, construct and analyze student tests, facilitate student learning of technology, prepare and present lectures and much more.

Partial Contents:
- Making Clinical Assignments
- Supervising a Clinical Group
- Designing a Learning Contract
- Teaching Students to Work in Groups
- Planning to Give a Lecture
- Planning a Successful Seminar
- Course Design, Implementation, and Evaluation
- Textbook and Reading Assignment Selection
- Designing and Grading a Major Assignment
- Designing and Grading a Minor Assignment
- Test Construction and Analysis
- Using Technology to Facilitate Learning
- Guiding Independent Study
- Helping Students Improve Writing Skills

2000 200pp 0-8261-6601-6 hard

536 Broadway, New York, NY 10012 • (212) 431-4370 • Fax (212) 941-7842
Order Toll-Free: 877-687-7476 • Order on-line: www.springerpub.com

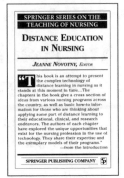